BODY BELLY SOUL

THE BLACK MOTHER'S GUIDE TO A PRIMAL, PEACEFUL, AND POWERFUL BIRTH

NICOLE BAILEY

© Copyright 2021 by Nicole Bailey. All rights reserved. No portion of this book may be reproduced, stored in a retrieval system, or transmitted in any form or by any means—electronic, mechanical, photocopy, recording, scanning, or other—except for brief quotations in critical reviews or articles, without the prior written permission of the publisher.

ISBN - 978-1-955090-16-2
ISBN for Ebook - 978-1-955090-17-9
Library of Congress Number: 2021918004

Cover design done by Samantha Jordan
https://www.sammijdesigns.com/

Copyediting by N. Amma Twum-Baah
https://www.ammaedits.com

DISCLAIMER

This book is intended to provide helpful and useful information. It is not intended to diagnose, treat, cure, or prevent any health problems or conditions, nor is it intended to replace the advice of a physician. No action should be taken solely on the contents of this book. Always consult your physician or a qualified health care provider on any matters regarding your health, and before adopting any suggestions in this book or drawing inferences from it.

The author and foreword author expressly disclaims any responsibility for any liability, loss, or risk, personal or otherwise, which is incurred consequently, directly, or indirectly, from the use and application of any of the contents of this book.

DEDICATION

For Alexandria, you are my biggest inspiration to equip and serve Black mothers and daughters who will follow in my footsteps. You give me passion and purpose.

For Johnny, my love, may we always fight inequality together and serve as an example in our community to promote change.

CONTENTS

FOREWORD 1

PREFACE 5

INTRODUCTION: THE FEAR AND CHALLENGES OF NATURAL BIRTH 9

PART 1: THE DECISION 25

    1: COMING TO TERMS WITH REALITY 27

    2: MAKING MY DECISION 34

PART 2: PREPARING TO FULLY AND SAFELY EXPERIENCE BIRTH ... 37

    3: DEVELOP YOUR MIND AND YOUR TRIBE 39

    4: FIND THE RIGHT PROVIDER AND LOCATION ... 46

    5: ASSEMBLE THE REST OF YOUR BIRTHING TEAM 68

    6: PREPARING YOUR BODY AND BELLY FOR DELIVERY 85

    7: CONNECT TO YOUR BABY AND YOUR SOUL 109

PART 3: WELCOME TO MOTHERHOOD 121

    8: POSTPARTUM PREPARATION AND CARE 123

9: BREASTFEEDING WHILE BLACK	139
10: ESTABLISHING A NEW NORMAL	160
ACKNOWLEDGMENTS	171
SOURCES CITED	173
ABOUT THE AUTHOR	179

FOREWORD

As a nurse with nearly 15 years of maternity care experience in hospital and community settings, I have witnessed the lack of Black voices being accepted on the topic discussed in *Body, Belly Soul*. Hospitals must meet goals, have quotas, and must make space for additional patients daily. Unfortunately, this pace in patient care can make hospital births seem like a factory, leading to unnecessary interventions that cause moms and babies undue stress and trauma. While caring for and speaking with moms and families postpartum, my experience is that they are often glad the birth experience is over, but do not feel like they had much input in how the process went. *Body, Belly, Soul* is here to change that narrative.

I met the author, Nicole Bailey, at a baby shower. As a healthcare professional focused on respectful maternal care, and Nicole having similar interests, we ended up chatting for hours. We bonded while discussing our potential journeys through motherhood and noticed that we had similar birth story expectations. We were both mothers passionate about reframing the birth experience for Black women, and we were both using our first-time pregnancies as an opportunity to educate ourselves by making conscious decisions on how we wanted our birthing experiences to go. Knowing that the birth experience can change in an instant, we were aware that we would have to accept some changes, while still holding true to our values. As a result of this preparation, we can now share positive stories about the joys of childbirth and the steps it takes to get there as an expectant mother.

A common thread Nicole and I also shared was having loving and supportive husbands and caring and courageous mothers throughout the process. If either of those is unavailable, we encourage women to create a strong support system of friends and/or relatives, who believe and feel the same way as she does about pregnancy and childbirth.

Seeing Nicole as a mother, so enthusiastic about the voices of minority mothers, reminds me that my role as a nurse is to advocate. When caring for my patients, especially those Black and Brown patients, I must listen to and respect their wishes, support them, and clarify their understanding of their current situations. Every birth story is different, but each deserves the same respect. As healthcare professionals, we attend to births every day, but to every mom and every family it is their unique individual experience and, treating it as just a number will not work.

I am writing this foreword during my second pregnancy, and *Body, Belly, Soul* reminds me that I have control over my birth experience and, as many chapters and sections of the book detail:

- I get to choose my provider and the location of delivery.
- I have a support system that I have chosen to be involved in.

- I control my thoughts with what I welcome into my ears, my mind, and my heart.
- I control the energy that I transfer to my baby.
- I control the ways I prepare my body for labor.
- I control the space where I will birth my baby.

With control, there comes the responsibility for me to make informed decisions. I must understand the entire process of what's happening to my body, belly, and my soul. I must begin by informing myself about the overall situation. This book will provide you with valuable questions to ask, decisions to ponder, and steps to take as you prepare for your birth experience. I can attest to the fact that *Body, Belly, Soul* gives you the necessary information, so you can stay in control of your birth story.

Dr. Lorraine Wilson Batts, DNP, RN

PREFACE

I imagine you picked up this book because current Black maternal statistics alarm you. Maybe you want an unmedicated birth but are unsure of how to start. Or you're the first one among your friends to become a mother and you have no idea what's next. If you are looking for positive narratives surrounding birth, or perhaps, you're a birth worker looking for ways to protect Black mothers, for whatever reason, whoever you are, I affirm you!

First, I want to commend you for taking the first step towards having a more enlightened birth experience. Whether you are expecting your first baby, your third baby, or simply guiding someone else through their pregnancy, taking interest in the Black birthing experience is the first step to reducing the current maternity statistics that are haunting the Black community.

We must ask ourselves, why are black mothers dying at a rate 3-4 times that of white women in the United States? That is 243% more likely to die from pregnancy and child-related complications. Lack of empathy from healthcare providers, the failure of health professionals to listen to the concerns of Black mothers, a perceived lesser value than our counterparts of other races, systemic racism in our healthcare systems, lack of providers who look like us, a lack of respect when it comes to Black women's expressions of pain, the habitual use of interventions, birthing by directions rather than instinct, overuse of our medical system, and so on. Sadly, the list goes on and on and one can say that this is history repeating itself or that nothing has changed at all.

So, how can we protect ourselves in maternity rooms when faced with a system that is so quick to reduce us to a statistic or an experiment? The answer is through preparation, advocating for ourselves, and raising our consciousness. Because the truth is that Black women are more likely to die during childbirth from interventions, and a robust preventative care plan will reduce the number of Black women finding themselves in need of higher levels of care resulting from complications. Only a small percentage of pregnancies initially fall into the category of complicated and require emergency services.

Birth requires that we prepare ourselves by focusing entirely on our mental, physical, and spiritual conditions. That we advocate, with the knowledge we have acquired through preparation, for the care that we deserve. This is done by becoming more conscious about the entire process and history of pregnancy, birthing, and postpartum, by taking a deep look into our ancestors' rituals and traditions. We will explore how to use formerly trusted ways of birthing in today's modern birth spaces, and how to arm ourselves with knowledge of all the stages of childbearing.

You have picked up this book because you plan on being intentional in preparations for your birthing experience. Your experience does not have to be unmedicated or fit into any definition of natural, but it should be accompanied by a more conscious mind, free of trauma, and must be momma-centered. Body Belly Soul seeks to promote the power of reconnecting to our roots, coupled with preparation and advocacy to promote more conscious birthing experiences. We will do this by filling you up with historic wisdom and the power to make instinctual decisions for you and your baby.

The thing about childbirth is that there is no way to know exactly how things will go. Each experience is uniquely different. Some women experience the exact labor they envisioned, whether that be a home birth or epidural-assisted hospital birth, while others are propelled into disoriented experiences with traumatic outcomes. Of course, this can happen to any woman, but the risks increase for women of color, and especially for Black women.

Now let's tap into why we need to focus on having more births that are primal, peaceful, and powerful!

INTRODUCTION:
THE FEAR AND CHALLENGES OF NATURAL BIRTH

Like many women today, I too had heard countless stories about the birthing process as a painful memory distorted by medication and fear. It took my mother sharing her birth story with me for me to realize that it only takes one story to move the needle (all puns intended). My mother's experience with childbirth for the first time was successful partly due to the support and love of my father. As my mother tells it, she was at a barbeque with my father on a warm spring night in May in a small German town outside of Wiesbaden, Germany, when she went into labor. My father took her to the local hospital and supported her throughout labor. She vividly recounts being supported by an elderly midwife and my father as her labor lasted throughout the night. While she labored, she walked the halls with my father through each contraction as he guided her breathing. My birth included no interventions. I was their firstborn, a baby girl, "a very peaceful baby", according to my mother. My mother has always been very intentional about sharing the fact that, back in her day, epidurals were nowhere near as common as they are today. She describes birth as something women were indeed born to do. Her sister, cousins, and her mother, my grandmother, all share common birth experiences, all of them having given birth without epidurals or requiring C-sections.

Today, nearly one in every three births is done by C-section. At least, these were the stats back in 2008. I can only imagine that the number is much higher today. That's 32% of births, according to the Annual Summary of Vital Statistics, a report from the National Center for Health Statistics, and the Johns Hopkins Bloomberg School of Public Health. Of the one in three births, Black mothers were most likely to birth their babies this way. And here's the kicker: "The rates are going up, but we are not improving the health of babies or moms," says George Macones, vice chairman of the American Congress of Obstetricians and Gynecologists (ACOG).

I became pregnant with my first child in 2019. I was excited and looking forward to the day when my baby girl would arrive. Almost immediately, I started to think about the journey of bringing my child into this world and what that journey would look like. I always desired to have a conscious birthing experience. This desire stemmed from my inherent connection to my ancestors who had birthed before me on this very soil, as well as my strong distaste for needles. To be honest, I feared the idea of needles, immobility, the insertion of a urine catheter, and relinquishing control more than birth itself. This fear of needles, injections, and IVs dating back to my childhood, quickly resurfaced when I attended my first few prenatal appointments, which required multiple blood tests and little transparency around standard prenatal visits. I quickly realized that I also had little trust in the US medical system. In my defense, there's not much to trust between the current statistics and the long-standing mistreatment of black bodies.

I have reflected on what my ancestors endured. When resources were limited or simply denied to people of color, and days were long and intense on southern plantations, where maternity leave was unheard of unless you were respected as a good breeding woman. I have heard stories of runaway slaves birthing in cotton fields attempting to seek refuge, while others worked until the last crop was picked and birthed in log cabins surrounded by granny midwives and kinfolk. I assure you, we once birthed with no interventions but with plenty of wisdom and intimacy. I have admired our tenacity for as long as I can remember. As a young girl, I was strangely intrigued by the stories of exploitation of Black women on southern plantations and how, despite their circumstances, the Black population continued to thrive against all odds. I carry this strength in my soul. This piqued my curiosity and boosted my confidence in pursuing a birthing experience that aligned with my beliefs. I believed that our bodies were created to birth and that a more conscious birth would be the journey I set out to pursue. I confirmed my intuition when my mother assured me that birth is a natural process, and I would indeed find the strength to follow through without interventions.

At the time that my mother told me about her experience with labor and delivery, she did not mention a small tear she sustained from pushing me out while lying on her back. It was after I had birthed my daughter on all fours that she shared this with me. I appreciate that my mother did not project a piece of her experience on me. She allowed me to have my own experience which resulted in an unmedicated birth with no tears. This is important because when women share their fears and pains surrounding birth, it prevents other women from properly preparing for their own experiences. In other words, we are perpetuating the FEAR. Passing down stories of caution rather than stories of strength. Instead, she reiterated that an unmedicated birth was highly achievable and that the most important thing was a supportive partner or team. Not only are those words true, but they are also one of the key factors in achieving a birth with minimal interventions. We will discuss later how important surrounding yourself with the proper birth team and tribe are.

HOW FEAR GIVES WAY TO MEDICATED BIRTHS

Fear is paralyzing. I'm sure we can all remember a moment when fear stopped or delayed us from pursuing something we wanted to achieve. Maybe you wanted to pursue a new passion, start a new career, or conquer your fear of heights but something held you back. When we allow fear to take over the body during labor, we're subconsciously telling the body not to move forward, subsequently invoking tension instead of relaxation. This causes our body to go into protection mode which then introduces the hormones associated with the notion of flight

> The most powerful element of fear is anticipation, when we hold onto fear, we are making room for our fears to develop.

or fight, epinephrine (adrenaline) and norepinephrine (noradrenaline). When these two hormones are released, the body perceives danger, and the stress and anxiety of pregnancy can elevate maternal stress hormones. Not only does this ultimately stop the progression of labor, but it also opens the window for medical interventions to be introduced. Approaching birth with fear is known to have detrimental long-term effects on babies, including impacts on brain development and stress responsiveness. I also want you to know that there's so much more to look forward to in your birth experience than focusing your attention on avoiding pain and manifesting fear. The most powerful element of fear is anticipation, when we hold onto fear, we are making room for our fears to develop.

The tension that is associated with focusing on fear and pain is exactly what inevitably leads to intense pain, a long list of interventions, and eventually a longer recovery. Epidurals cannot change this, only our thoughts and minds can. As stated in the law of thermodynamics, energy is neither created nor destroyed. Energy can only be transferred or changed from one form to another. So, while epidurals may postpone or transfer that energy, it will inevitably show up elsewhere. In the case of birth, it often slows down labor and prolongs the birthing experience. I will discuss more in Chapter 7, Connecting to your Soul and Baby about how to dispel thoughts of fear and pain.

This is how it works. Epidurals can beneficially reduce maternal pain and epinephrine levels, which may have been inhibiting labor. However, the rapid drop in epinephrine can contribute to hypertension and uterine hyperstimulation. In many cases, contractions reduce over time because oxytocin also decreases. Reductions in both epinephrine-norepinephrine and oxytocin with an epidural can contribute to a prolonged pushing stage and assisted vaginal birth. Epidurals do not decrease stress hormones; they may increase them in labor, increasing the risk of a cesarean section due to fetal distress. Let us not forget the secondary issues associated with epidurals, such as temporary paralysis, a lack of sensation in the body, the inability to walk or squat during labor, longer recovery periods, having to insert a urine catheter, and the inability to push in sync with the baby and contractions. As a result of these numerous effects, the epidural often backfires on the laboring mother and slows down labor.

Once a doctor diagnoses a woman as "failing to progress," he or she will introduce Pitocin through an intravenous insertion to make contractions more intense and speed things along. Pitocin is an artificial hormone that acts similarly to oxytocin but does not have the same love/bonding effect as the actual hormone oxytocin. The intense and faster contractions cause the baby to become distressed (i.e., in a panic over the exacerbation of contractions caused by Pitocin and low heart rate due to the back-to-back interventions), which then causes the mother to be informed that an emergency C-section is necessary for the safety of the distressed baby. Because a mother's priority is the safety of her baby, she feels she has no choice but to agree to a C-section to save her unborn baby, even if she planned to have a vaginal birth. This creates a false narrative; the doctor appears as the hero that saved the baby when this entire process may have been avoided by simply introducing fewer interventions and letting the natural birth process play out. While I understand that this may not be everyone's story and, of course, there are valid medical reasons for a C-section, this is indeed one of the most common and preventable cycles experienced in modern birthing spaces. We all have a friend, sister, auntie, or cousin, whose story went exactly like that. And more than likely, due to their memory lapse and lack of birth education, they left out the determining factor: that they were induced or given Pitocin, which led things down that path. The truth is that hospital systems are crafting a narrative that leaves women feeling disoriented, desperate, and overwhelmed. Hospital staff is typically aware of the ripple effects caused by medical interventions. They know that inducing or administering certain medications, will cause a ripple effect and, more than likely, reduce the baby's heart rate, but they neglect to share this information with mothers. All this goes to show that Black mothers are not given the right to full consent but are instead coerced to agree to terms or circumstances that we think our bodies created.

Since the 1970s, C-section rates among women have increased from 5% to 30% with no decrease in the infant or maternal mortality rates. This is a clear indication that C-sections are not only happening when necessary but also as an effect of the habitual intervention cycle used in hospitals across the country. The World Health Organization advises against the C-section rates rising above 10-15% in an industrialized country because higher rates expose mother and baby to undue risks.

In 2015, Dr. Amanishakete Ani, a psychologist who lectures across the country about Black liberation and the systemic oppression that affects the daily lives of Black people in the United States, wrote a publication in the Journal of African American Studies entitled *C-Section and Racism: Cutting into the Heart of the Black Family*. In the publication, Dr. Ani unveiled the insidious and deep contours of social regulation associated with the practice of "cutting" which is inherent to the longstanding practice of regulating Black women's reproductive capabilities. Given the glaringly uneven rates of C-sections among Black women, Ani explains the importance of gaining knowledge of traditional and ancient birthing practices, knowing all the risks associated with this method of birthing, and recognizing the intrinsic racism in the elemental levels of our lives. In her assessment, she identifies Cesarean sections as being like other forms of "existential violence" such as police brutality, fraternal murder, and mass incarceration directed at Black people. She characterizes these phenomena as "tentacles" of a larger political entity whereby they function to consistently contain life and impede the endurance of Black communities. Ani argues that the dramatic increase and ongoing overuse of cesarean sections as a method of delivery among Black women are "driven by a continuing history of commoditized oppression and exploitation on physical terms."

MODERN WOMEN AND THE RISE IN MEDICATED BIRTHS

People attribute my ability to have had an unmedicated birth to my presumed high tolerance for pain. I ask, "high tolerance where?" I have experienced no surgeries; I have no tattoos and the most basic piercings. I hate roller coasters and I am in no way a daredevil. I followed my intuitions. These intuitions led me to prepare my body, belly, and soul. I put fear aside and was able to move through labor with strength. This strength gave me autonomy over my birthing experience. My birth was free of interventions. This led to controlled, manageable labor and graceful recovery. This is something I achieved not only through physical and mental preparation but by manifestation also. By visualizing the entire process of giving birth, when the time came, my body did not fight, it did exactly what I had spent months envisioning. I was able to release fear and welcome strength, allowing my body to release a free flow of oxytocin, beta-endorphins, prolactin, and catecholamines hormones to do their biological magic. These four powerful and natural hormones come together to create a beautiful symphony during the most organic birthing experience. Oxytocin causes labor contractions and helps create feelings of love, calmness, and connection to others. Beta-endorphins relieve stress and pain around the time of birth. Prolactin, also called the "mothering hormone," has many roles, one of which includes producing breast milk. Catecholamines help you and your baby feel alert and ready for birth and protect your baby's heart and brain during strong labor contractions. The hormonal physiology of childbearing has evolved over millions of years to optimize reproductive success through our bodies. Women were created with reproduction as a function of their bodies, so know that you have everything you need before you choose to enter a hospital.

Due to an abundance of societal pressures, birth does not happen as spontaneously in modern times as it once did. Now, it must be an intentional decision. It was not a coincidence that I experienced a gentle birth experience, it was my intention, my preparation, my willingness to take control and release all fear. I took guidance from confident women who had birthed before me, whose knowledge and enlightenment allowed me to listen to and trust my body. I purposely probed like-minded women for their stories and carried those stories with me during my journey. I manifested the exact birth I envisioned for myself and my family, while deliberately rejecting stories and providers who projected pain, fear, and loss of control.

Modern birth has benefitted from many medical advances, and from highly skilled and committed maternity care providers, especially for mothers and babies who require special care. However, the current high rates of maternity care interventions surpass the actual need and pose a detriment to the healthy majority. These interventions are creating a narrative that says women are not capable of birthing their babies without medical attention. Generally, the most effective way to avoid interventions and C-sections is by choosing mother-centered care providers and birth locations. Not the mother. The provider. The provider is altering the outcomes. Yet, when expecting mothers are being told that they need a C-section, it is because the baby is in distress, but who and what caused this baby to be in distress?

There have been a few books written regarding the importance of removing fear and following our womanly instincts from birth dating back to 1959. The Holy Grail of natural childbirth books is *Childbirth Without Fear*, written by Grantly Dick-Read. His primary goal was to restore the art of natural childbirth, and he is regarded as the one responsible for the household term "Natural Childbirth."

> Black Women were once supported by sisters, aunties and neighbors who supported them emotionally, physically, and spiritually through their birthing journey.

According to Grantly,

> "Healthy childbirth was never intended by the natural law to be painful. Normally, birth is carried out by natural processes from beginning to end, influenced by natural emotions and perfected by the harmony of the mechanism [with the woman] conscious throughout the progress of her baby's birth, so that she can truly fulfill herself emotionally when she sees and welcomes the child emerging from her womb into the world". Natural childbirth also meant that the baby "is not separated from its mother and placed in a communal nursery. That she can have her husband with her during her baby's birth."
>
> - Grantly Dick-Read

> We can save a generation of Black mothers by reaching back into our roots and reexploring the power of storytelling.

Read also expands on how this art of childbirth was lost as the Modern Woman and modern obstetric practices came to the forefront. Remember that this book was written in the 1950s. Since then, we have only grown to become more modern and out of touch with the birthing process. We are *Modern Women*! We have so much more on our plates than the sole duty of rearing children. We are not as active as our ancestors were, spending 8 hours a day standing on their feet working on a southern plantation or as household nannies. No, we spend those same 8 hours behind our screens, being mostly sedentary. And we are accomplishing great things as business owners, CEOs, managing households, and navigating corporate jobs and side hustles. Oh, yes, we are, yet to experience one of our most primal activities, we will need to tap into a different mindset. This modern era contributes to our struggle to slow down and tap into our most basic instincts to experience the miracle of life. The medical industry exposed this void and has been able to replace it with interventions, fear, and medical expenses, with the average C-section costing anywhere up to $22K compared to $11.5K for vaginal deliveries. This is one benefit of exploitation hospitals are gaining from misleading more Black mothers into needing a C-section. The current situation stands that by handing over our power and knowledge of birth, we have seen a deliberate increase in deaths, and traumatic and disconnected childbirth experiences of Black mothers and babies. I'm writing this book out of concern for the Black birthing experience and the desire to see an increase in healthy and connected birth experiences amongst us.

I want to be the story to you that my mom was to me, the story that sparks interest and encourages you to take more control over your birthing experience from the very beginning through to the very end when you're holding your baby close, and nursing and bonding because you rejected fear. Unfortunately, the stories I've heard from many women had a common thread. That common thread was that they all lacked interest or time in preparing for childbirth. Many of them were strong, intelligent, career-driven women who, while trying to balance it all, decided to fall for the age-old myth that epidurals would be their safety net. They were sisters who failed to take birthing classes, decided against hiring a doula, and didn't dare to switch providers. As much as I love these women, when I reflect on the steps they missed, I can't help but wonder whether there could have been a more connected experience.

Historically, it was common practice for all women to have witnessed many births before going through their own. Black Women were once supported by sisters, aunties, and neighbors who supported them emotionally, physically, and spiritually through their birthing journey. These women were able to offer a great degree of wisdom, reassurance, and experience.

I believe that we can save a generation of Black mothers by reaching back into our roots and reexploring the power of storytelling. My purpose is to simultaneously pay homage to our ancestors while protecting and providing a solution for our future. We need to reduce our dependence on the very patriarchal system that does not keep women's health and reproduction at the forefront, much less Black women's. I want this book to be a reminder that we can still pass down knowledge and comfort as we once did to our expecting sister. Warning against the common storylines that are perpetuated in birth spaces from early arrivals, inductions, and lack of advocacy, while encouraging our fellow sisters to strip themselves of the fear and fall into the miracle and beauty of birth.

In this book, I take you along my purposeful journey of preparation while shedding light on the intentional steps you can take to increase your odds of an unmedicated birth and to have a more informed birthing experience. Throughout my pregnancy, I prepared like I was training for the Olympics and studying for the MCATs. I watched documentaries to understand the process of birth. I switched providers once I realized how significant of an impact care providers can have on a woman's freedom to birth the way she wants to. I interviewed doulas. I found a prenatal yoga class and other safe prenatal exercises that I practiced daily. I used language unique to me to describe labor pains and pressures. I will admit that some of this obsession over preparation came from anxiety and the eagerness to be over prepared rather than underprepared. But I also had a strong desire to bring my firstborn into this world as a healthy and thriving baby. I intended to give her the most powerful start that I could, beginning with a flourishing pregnancy and a harmonious birth.

By the end of this book, I want you to know that preparation and knowledge have an impact on your ability to birth confidently and puts you in charge of decisions affecting you and your baby in the delivery room. I also want you to know that you are not dependent on the systems that seek to exploit you. You are free to make more conscious decisions surrounding your birth experiences, leading to a more enlightened and connected being for you and your baby. Know that birthing is a spectrum, and you may land anywhere on that spectrum depending on various variables, but the most important place to be is involved and aware. This is how we, you and I, and every Black mother in the United States, can disrupt the current state of Black maternity in this country.

The way we birth our babies is going to be the way that we parent and the way that we live. To raise our children safely, we must recognize that the foundation we lay sets the tone for a safer world to live in. I'm here to show you how to prepare, make informed decisions, and empower yourself to move in the best interests of your unborn baby and yours; let's keep going to see how.

PART 1:
THE DECISION

The maternal mortality rate of a nation is an indicator of its general health. In the United States, the maternal mortality rate is worse today than it was 25 years ago. Among these disturbing statistics are

> "When you change the way you view birth, the way you birth will change."
> — Marie F. Morgan, founder of HypnoBirthing

Black women who are dying from pregnancy complications and childbirth at an alarming rate in preventable situations. As a result, a time that should be reserved for the joys of new life and rebirth is now plaguing Black women with fears of complications and uncertainty. Every day, we're struck by a news story or statistic highlighting the recent acknowledgment of neglect on the prenatal and postnatal care of the Black woman. Take celebrities such as Beyonce and Serena Williams for example. These women are not only in the best shape of their lives but also have access to unlimited resources. and yet, they still found themselves in a maternity crisis that nearly killed them. Serena Williams is a great example when it comes to being conscious of your own body, informed about your medical history, and advocating for the care you know you need. We should all strive for this type of trust in ourselves.

Subsequently, this also shows us that regardless of socioeconomic status, educational level, or household income, all Black women are at a significantly higher risk for medical neglect than white women.

1

COMING TO TERMS WITH REALITY

This is by no means the first time we have found the Black family under attack in this country. The traditional understanding of reproductive freedom has blatantly denied Black women, in this country, control over critical decisions about their bodies since slavery. Now, more than ever, we need to take a deeper dive into the importance of reclaiming our

> Our country is thriving off the miseducation and manipulation of black and brown bodies. It's time for us to acknowledge what is happening, take a stand for ourselves and create sustainable Black communities that make informed health decisions for our own future.

bodies and minds surrounding our birth decisions. The denial of Black reproductive autonomy serves the interests of white supremacy and American capitalism from the conception of this country. Why do we continue to trust a system that was not built to protect us or see us strive? Let's face it, our country is thriving off the miseducation and manipulation of black and brown bodies. It is time for us to acknowledge what is happening, take a stand for ourselves, and create sustainable Black communities that make informed health decisions for our future. We can achieve this by starting where it counts the most—by choosing providers who look like us and who listen to us, and by reducing our dependence on doctors and hospitals in the case of low-risk pregnancies. We all have a position in this revolution, mine is to nurture and empower Black mothers to return to holistic choices, to change the narrative for our future generations, and to promote more positive outcomes for our birth stories. By reaching for a more instinctual birth experience, your mind will be more open to holistic practices. Also, you will organically become more informed and aware of the systemic oppression occurring in our healthcare system.

Studies have shown time and time again that the cause of the disparity in health for Black birthing mothers and babies has little to do with poverty and poor lifestyle habits. Education and income have been proven to offer little protection. A Black woman with an advanced degree is more likely to lose her baby than a white woman with less than an eighth-grade education," according to New York Times contributor, Linda Villarosa, in an article she titled, "Why America's Black Mothers and Babies Are in a Life-or-Death Crisis."

The systematic, institutionalized denial of reproductive freedom has uniquely marked Black women's history in America. Considering this—from slave masters' economic stake in bonded women's fertility to the racist strains of early birth control policy to sterilization abuse of Black women during the

1960s and 1970s to the most recent campaign to inject Norplant and Depo-Provera in the arms of Black teenagers and welfare mothers—paints a powerful picture of the link between race and reproductive freedom in America. The use of legal means to legitimize and standardize racist practices comes as no surprise. The reproduction rights of Black women have been under surveillance, used at the disposal of slave holders, the government, and medical industries since 1808 when the United States stopped importing slaves.

Here is a convincing list of reasons why many Black people in the United States do not trust the medical industry with their reproduction and maternal health. These stories should serve as cautious reminders when it comes to the importance of choosing healthcare providers who look like you, while advocating for yourself in all settings but especially those associated with the procreation of Black lives.

The Tuskegee Syphilis Experiment - Also known as the "Tuskegee Study of Untreated Syphilis in the Negro Male." This study involved over 600 men and 399 of those men were diagnosed with syphilis but instead of being treated and informed of this diagnosis, they were told they had bad blood and left untreated. Once treatment was available, these men were still not treated which resulted in death, exposure to families, blindness, and other ailments due to disease progression. This experiment on Black men went on for 40 years. Forty years of manipulation, experimentation, and unfair treatment ending in the genocide of a whole black community of fathers in Macon County, Alabama.

Norplant for welfare mothers and teens in Baltimore - In the early 1990s, Black welfare mothers and Black high school teen girls were targeted for Norplant insertions primarily to control the reproduction of black poverty without proper informed consent. Norplant was the first subdermal implantable device that prevented pregnancy for 5 years. Welfare women were forced and financially manipulated into using Norplant. Once implanted, however, doctors ignored complaints from these women and refused to remove the implants. A private 200k grant awarded to Baltimore City for health and education prompted access to Norplant in primarily Black middle and high schools, waiving parental consent.

Reproductive surgery experimentation on enslaved Black women – To some, Dr. Sims is known as the father of gynecology, but his road to this honor is not an admirable one. His discoveries and findings were done at the expense of enslaved Black women in Alabama without anesthesia and their consent. After many years as a plantation physician, he moved his medical practice to New York City where he opened a women's hospital for White women and conducted the same procedures on them using anesthesia. He claimed that Black women don't feel pain.

Sterilization of Black women and young girls in North Carolina - The Eugenics Board of North Carolina (EBNC) was a Board in North Carolina formed, in July 1933, by the North Carolina State Legislature by the passage of House Bill 1013, entitled 'An Act to Amend Chapter 34 of the Public Laws of 1929 of North Carolina Relating to the Sterilization of Persons Mentally Defective'. The targets of that board's 45-year reign were disproportionately Black and female, and almost universally poor. They included victims of rape and incest and women who were already mothers, as well as their daughters. The state's remedy for all of them was forced or coerced sterilization. It has been stated that eugenic sterilization was an attempt to control the reproduction of women on welfare.

The disenfranchisement of Black midwives and doulas - Black women's accomplishments and contributions have often been overlooked in US history, and the journey of bringing midwifery to the US is no different. The art of midwifery owes much of its affluence to Black midwives. Midwifery was primarily a tradition amongst Black women, dating back to pre-colonization in African villages and communities. During this period, midwives supported their communities as family counselors, breastfeeding consultants, postpartum doulas, nutritionists, and family planning counselors. They were birth advocates who provided holistic resources and care for their people.

This rich tradition was passed down from healer to healer and practiced even during slavery. When doctors lacked prioritization or understanding of slave mothers during pregnancy, it was midwives who provided care with the resources that they had. Many times, babies ended up being born at the hands of a trusted community midwife. Let us also not forget that these midwives were themselves being held captive and performed such intricate care while under the most severe conditions. Of importance is also the fact that Black midwives not only provided care for their fellow slaves, but they provided prenatal care and midwifery services to their slave masters' wives.

After the Civil War, obstetrics and gynecology emerged and sought to discredit midwives, leading to the outlaw and heavy reduction of Black midwives. Although midwives have reemerged, they are often not women of color, the practice is now more widely used by non-blacks, and faces heavy scrutiny. It can be difficult in certain southern states to obtain insurance coverage, making the use of midwives now a luxury and a privilege. These women were once disgraced for the cultural and holistic ideals to uplift the credibility of obstetrics and gynecology. I encourage my fellow birthing sisters, to refer midwives and doulas of color and to advocate for the resurgence of birthing our way as a key factor in preserving our community. I also champion for my young sisters to go into these professions and flood these industries for our protection. Step into these places knowing your history and aim to revive our traditions, even if that is to simply encourage birthing mothers to educate and trust themselves.

My Grandfather was born in 1937 in Fayetteville, North Carolina, he was the oldest of 9 children. As part of my research for this book, I asked him about his birth story and who delivered him and all eight of his siblings. "My grandmother," he simply replied. And then he continued, "Oh, Nicole, back in my day, we didn't go to hospitals for births. Whenever my mother, your Grandma Joe, was nearly due with any one of her nine children, she would head down to the "Big House," just another name for my grandmother's house. She was responsible for birthing everyone in the family. She was well-known for caring for women during this time."

To hear that my very own great-great-grandmother was a midwife brought me so much joy. Birth was indeed once a protected experience. An intimate encounter that happened at home, amongst trusted family members. You knew exactly who they were responsible for birthing before you, they knew your family history and I'm sure they weren't rushing or interfering with the birth process.

2

MAKING MY DECISION

In villages, across islands, and on plantations, we once birthed our children and continued to grow our families under exceedingly difficult circumstances while having very connected birth experiences.

After navigating through our complex maternal history and gaining a better understanding of common maternity ward narratives, I felt empowered to trust my body and to lean on the combination of my newly acquired knowledge and intuition while being at peace with bringing my baby earth-side. I envisioned laboring at home for as long as possible in the comfort of my own home, with the assistance of a midwife and a doula and with the man I chose to go on this journey with. And that is exactly what we did. I leaned into this strength from our ancestors and deeply believed in the possibility of my own birthing experience by being surrounded with affirming love and comfort from my village.

I now know that for centuries, Black women took pride in the responsibility of providing emotional, physical and cultural support, and it assured me that hiring a doula was going to be a vital step in my preparation. I found that my hesitation towards traditional medical practices aligns me more with the fundamental practices of midwifery, as they are known to encourage more holistic approaches before relying on modern medical practices. The most common way to avoid a C-section is by paying attention to your choice of provider, the location of your delivery, and the continuous support given by a doula. We will discuss more in "Choosing your Provider," and "Developing Your Birth Tribe." There's great power in stories being shared amongst women because we do not know what someone does not share. When positive birth experiences are kept quiet, it only amplifies the birth stories that were guided with fear and pain leading to an increase of interventions for all women. I want to remind women that positive births *are* experienced. Every labor story is not filled with emergency medical waivers. As a matter of fact, birth can be undoubtedly beautiful, empowering, and gentle if we reduce the number of interventions used. Yes, birth can be gentle! What I've found from sitting down with numerous Black mothers and from my personal experience is that the key lies in taking control of your experience from the very beginning. Becoming a Black mother in this country with our history and access to information can be overwhelming and frightening. This is a guide to help you prepare and to remind you of what is possible when you surround yourself with positive thoughts, beliefs, and possibilities of labor.

I have found that correlations between the lack of knowledge and empowerment are a significant driver in the outcomes for our Black mothers. Most importantly, we need more empowering stories being shared amongst women of color and to be equipped with the tools we need to regain control over our birthing experiences. Black women of childbearing age need more relatable peer support and I want to ensure that starts now.

Throughout the rest of this book, I will explain the steps I took to prepare for my intervention-free birthing experience, unveil some more historical context, and share some healing techniques that I found beneficial. I'm not here to shame any woman's journey or experience, but I do hope that this allows the seasoned mother to reflect on her experience and share that as a benchmark as well. The power of sharing stories amongst our community will ensure that no mother feels alone during this transformative time. Even if your birth story has a different ending, you will find that preparing your body for the most organic experience will give you the knowledge to advocate for yourself in any birth situation. Often, we are told that if the baby is healthy, it does not matter what the mother endures, I want to counter that because your journey as a mother doesn't end the day your baby is born, it's the day it begins. This day will have an impact on your postpartum recovery, breastfeeding journey, the story you share with the next mother, and most importantly yourself!

This is not a week-by-week guide. This is my birth preparation journey. It is the journey of how I prepared myself to experience the birth of my firstborn fully and safely. Come along with me, let's journey through this together.

PART 2:
PREPARING TO FULLY AND SAFELY EXPERIENCE BIRTH

You just found out that you're pregnant and you've picked up a copy of this book. What now? I would suggest that you start by envisioning your positive birthing experience.

> Giving birth should be your greatest achievement, not your greatest fear.
> —Jane Weiderman

Where are you? Who is there? What sounds do you hear? What birthing tools are you using? Is there water involved? Close your eyes and visualize giving birth. Do you see a sensual water birth with your partner supporting you physically and emotionally? Do you envision a strong doula who has empowered many women to achieve their goal of unmedicated labor? Do you envision a birth in the comfort of your own home with the ones you love? All of these are possible.

As with most major decisions, you need to be informed and intentional. It is time to become better acquainted with the birthing process and learn the language. This is easier now than ever before with full birthing videos being posted on social media, doula docu-series, and podcasts of many women sharing their birth stories. These mediums of viewing birth have made the birthing experience more relatable and obtainable. There is nothing like seeing your favorite blogger birth like a champ! In this age of technology, you can see and watch any type of labor and delivery you want on almost any platform, Facebook, YouTube, even Netflix. This will set the tone for your birth. Keep in mind that the stories you consume have a major impact on your philosophies and possibilities surrounding birth. So, pick mediums and content that remove fear and pain from the birthing process.

3

DEVELOP YOUR MIND AND YOUR TRIBE

When I was pregnant with my firstborn, I watched only peaceful home births accompanied by supportive partners, a reassuring doula, and a midwife as the medical professional. I was so enamored with the idea of water birth, I spent most of my pregnancy watching water birth videos and planning for one. Unfortunately, the hospital where I had planned to give birth was in the process of replacing its tubs throughout my pregnancy. But even though my birth experience fell a bit short of the birth plan I had originally envisioned, I can confidently say that I only consumed birth content that showed women in control of their bodies, taking their time to push, and being symphonious with their babies. These images were able to guide me through my own birthing process. This control comes from knowledge and the elimination of fear. I noticed that these women did not fear the process, and they trusted and listened to their bodies. We will discuss how being present and at peace plays a major factor in your birthing experience in Chapter 7 (Connect to Your Baby and Your Soul).

Next, I consulted with like-minded Black and Brown women about the resources and tools they used to ensure their own birthing experiences were achieved. What I found was that it is common for women who view birth as a natural process to have birth supported by midwives instead of doctors. And as I surrounded myself with more mothers and expecting mothers, I discovered what birth outcomes each local hospital was known for. My current hospital at the time was known for C-sections!

One mother suggested that I watch a documentary by Ricki Lake and Abby Epstein called *The Business of Being Born*. The documentary follows Ricki's homebirth journey with her second baby due to some unsettling feelings she had with her first hospital birth. *The Business of Being Born* heavily examines how the American healthcare system approaches childbirth. The traditional form of births in the U.S. involves hospitals, drugs, and obstetricians, while births in many other countries utilize midwives and are far less medicalized. The documentary uncovers the realities of maternity care in this country where obstetricians are considered the standard of maternity care. According to the documentary, due to their strong surgical training, many obstetricians have never even seen birth in its most natural state in medical school. Instead, they are studying the transaction of surgical and intervention births. They have never seen life unveil in its purest form. Therefore, they are entering birth spaces where there is a lack of trust in the capabilities of women's bodies and where they are not fully competent to assist women in search of a more instinctual experience. The documentary also focuses on the fact that hospitals are businesses that thrive on quick turnovers, the use of drugs to induce and speed up labor, and filling and emptying beds at a faster rate.

I cannot stress enough the importance of surrounding yourself with informed and positive mothers who not only want a healthy birthing experience for you but also respect what you want your birthing story to be. Primarily, the system is just that. A system. It has perfected the art of ensuring women are stripped of the courage to choose their path. As you draw closer to the day, reinforcement from these same women (who will become your tribe) will be vital to you remaining motivated. In my corner, I had these wonderful sisters who were positive influences in my birthing preparation.

Earth Mama is my deeply rooted Mama, well connected with her ancestors, her spirit, and her baby. She's located in LA. She explained to me that she went to the water to summon her ancestors' guidance to induce her labor the week her baby was due. She knows all the natural remedies for producing more milk. If you tell her your milk supply is low, she will give you five natural herbs to pick from the local herbalist. She is still breastfeeding her beautiful baby girl at 2 years old, and she speaks with such great wisdom. Earth Mama is the big sister I never had. She advised me to give birth on all 4's, which I did naturally.

When I asked Earth Mama why she decided to have an unmedicated birth, this is how she responded: "I consider all births to be natural, but I chose for my birth experience to be vaginal with no drugs because I don't trust the hospital for Black women. I believe the human body is capable of doing it on its own if given the freedom to move freely." Although there were times when she wanted to speed up her labor, she felt her experience with her husband, midwife, and doula was phenomenal.

She felt supported and her birth plan was followed and most importantly respected.

Anchored/Balance Mama is my super chic, calm, and collected mama. She is extremely down-to-earth but a tad bit glamorous. Our babies were due less than 3 weeks apart. We moved providers together and discussed all our grievances surrounding the OB/GYN process. She birthed before me and reassured me that I was prepared and that I would knock this out of the park. And I did! I swear, once she told me that I would, I knew I could do it. It was not as if she had birthed years ago. She birthed yesterday and we pretty much followed all the same preparation. Her water broke right before it was time to push and guess what? Mine did too!

When I asked her why she decided to have an unmedicated birth, she shared this:

"I initially decided to have an unmedicated birth because I was very afraid of needles, and the idea of being partially paralyzed terrified me. I never considered an epidural necessary for childbirth and I heard that other pain medication measures weren't highly effective. I wouldn't describe myself as someone with a "high pain tolerance," but I knew an unmedicated birth was something I could certainly handle." She birthed with both a midwife and a doula after deciding to part ways with a popular Washington, D.C.-based OB/GYN practice at 16 weeks. "Although I liked her, I could tell that the culture of the practice wasn't right for me. Interventions were the standard there, at all stages of the process. Also, they deliver at the hospital with the highest C-Section rate in the area." She describes her birth as, "smooth, naturally progressive, and calm. "It was single-handedly the best day of my life!"

Mommy Blogger is my NYC mommy blogger and glorified working mama! She's up to speed on all things that ease the transition into motherhood and how to seamlessly do it all while looking fabulous. Although I have known her for maybe 15 years, motherhood brought us closer together. I was pregnant with my first while she was pregnant with her second. Right before I was due, she shared a very intimate video of her laboring with her firstborn, supported by her doula and loving husband. This was the only video I had seen of someone I knew giving birth, so it meant everything to me that she shared it.

When I asked her why she decided to have an unmedicated birth, she shared this: "When I became pregnant, my friend Amber gave me a book titled, *Supernatural Childbirth* by Jackie Mize. It inspired me to trust my body to successfully bring my babies into this world naturally. I also watched *The Business of Being Born* and realized that I didn't want any interventions to possibly interfere with my God-given ability to bring my babies into the world. My birth experiences were amazing. I felt like they were an out-of-body experience. After I delivered my son (my first) I didn't remember much. I just remembered being in this place, this space of Zen and tranquility. It truly was beautiful. I don't remember the pain; I just remember the deep breathing and excitement. It was a fairytale delivery.

With my second, I had some complications. She was a week past her due date and my fluids were incredibly low. I had prodromal labor for about two weeks. These are not Braxton Hicks contractions, but real contractions that just never progress. They wanted to induce me on my due date but let me go a few days past. I finally had a night full of contractions that were not prodromal and went to the hospital to deliver. They told me because of my low fluids that I needed to be admitted to the hospital that day. They were pushing for interventions, but we settled on allowing them to break my water (which they did twice because so little fluids came out that they thought the first time was unsuccessful). I was still able to bring my baby into this world safely and without medication- that is a blessing!

Overall, childbirth made me feel like a superhero. That no matter what, my body did exactly what I commanded of it and what I prayed over it to do. Birth can be traumatic if it isn't done with intent, knowledge, and love. I am just grateful that my stories are what they are - I recognize that this isn't the case for all mamas.

These three women were my preparation and postpartum tribe. They shared their powerful unmedicated birth stories with me and affirmed that women that look like me were indeed more than capable of a positive, healthy, and peaceful birth experience. They knew the power of affirming me and each sent me into the birth space with a piece of their wisdom. They shared how they avoided interventions, how they conquered contraction hurdles, how they kept calm, and when they knew it was time to push. I was able to pull so many gems and most importantly strength from these women.

PREPARE THE MIND AND TRIBE CHECKLIST:

- [ ] Watch birthing videos that reflect how I want to experience birth.
- [ ] Watch birthing documentaries to familiarize yourself with current medical practices and what to beware of
- [ ] Find a provider who advocates for the birth you desire.
- [ ] Assemble your birthing team.
- [ ] Hire a doula.
- [ ] Productive doula meetings
- [ ] Attend classes: birth, newborn, breastfeeding classes.
- [ ] Review birth plan
- [ ] Surround yourself with mothers who can share empowering stories.

4

FIND THE RIGHT PROVIDER AND LOCATION

I began attending my prenatal appointments with my initial obstetrician (OB/GYN). I had already begun researching and learning about the birthing process, so I arrived at each appointment excited and ready to discuss and share my new findings, only to leave feeling unheard and out of place. Pregnancy is supposed to be an exciting time for a new mom, but instead, it felt like business as usual, and not in a good way. As far as information and transparency were concerned, I didn't feel like I was being informed during my visits. I remember arriving at appointments without any overview of what to expect that day and encountering staff who spoke to me as if I had been on this journey before. What got on my final nerve was an incident that occurred when I told my obstetrician that I desired to have a natural birth. She looked at me and laughed. "Your first labor? Ha!" That was all she said. Let me mention that she was a Black woman. That broke my spirit! We are encouraged to birth with people who look like us, but the sad truth is that medical professionals who look like us are trained by the very system that is supporting the traumatic experiences we face as Black mothers. I realized that this practice and physician did not align with my ideology regarding birth and knew that it was time to start looking at other options. Had I continued seeing this OB/GYN who was comfortable with disregarding my birth plan, I knew for certain that I would have found myself in less than a favorable birthing situation.

This is why I urge you to listen to yourself and adhere to the signs from the very beginning. Many women fear switching providers because they often don't think it's worth the trouble, so they stay with their OB/GYN. You should know that switching providers, due to either fear of discrimination or because you feel unheard, is part of advocating for yourself and all future Black mothers. When you do so, you are drawing attention to unacceptable practices and protecting your family. It is never too late or early to make the best decision for you and your baby. My heart slowly breaks every time a mother tells me that she didn't follow her gut and switch providers. Or that even though she did not get the experience she had imagined; she was too busy or too tired to find a new provider.

Four months into my pregnancy, and on the heels of that last prenatal experience, I decided that I was going to explore midwives and hospital alternatives. I felt that having a midwife-supported birth better aligned with my history as a Black woman and my cautious approach to the medical industry, as well as my trust in the birthing process. Although I deeply longed for a homebirth, I deferred that dream until I had some experience under my belt. I quickly got to work looking for a way forward.

Here are the steps I took to transition my care to a midwife:

- I attended the midwife's information session at a slightly progressive academic hospital – where they explained more about the methodology surrounding midwifery practice and keeping women at the center of the birthing process. They explained the importance of embracing the steps in preparation for a more intervention-free birth. Pain medication was not something that was quickly offered, instead, they led with more holistic approaches.
- I set up a consultation to ensure that I was a good candidate. A proper review of medical records, ultrasound, and blood work is done to ensure you are considered a low-risk pregnancy.
- I requested a transfer of my medical records from my former OB/GYN, although there was a sense of unsettlement and burden from the staff. I reminded myself that this was my pregnancy and my process, and I had every right to choose the provider that was the best fit for me.

The midwives' information session made the birth I envisioned seem more obtainable. Their records included low C-sections and epidural rates, and a focus on uplifting mothers. Once I started with the midwife practice, I was given a full overview of what to expect at each visit, resources for preparation, and new parenthood. It was such a different feeling from what I had experienced at the OB/GYN's office. I felt heard and reminded that I was on a rite of passage to bring forth the miracle of life. To help you make a fully informed and conscious decision, I have laid out the history of both OB/GYN and Midwives. While both options serve as a valid support to ensure that your baby is delivered safely, know that when choosing your provider, you may very well be choosing your birth experience. Your choice of provider alters the odds of the birth you will have, will contribute to the number of interventions you have, and will reflect in the outcomes. Choosing the right provider is half the battle and one of the most important decisions you will make on this journey. It is like choosing your spouse. Prioritize finding a provider whose philosophies align with your vision for your birth experience. Remember that you are hiring a provider to support you, not to control you. You have ownership over your body and choices. When we are placed in birth spaces where medical professionals are controlling the narrative and focused on their metrics, we tend to lose track of our options and neglect maternal instincts.

THE HISTORY OF OBSTETRICS AND GYNECOLOGY

I don't know who needs to read this, but controlling your body is your human right. This is a right that has a deep-rooted historic context as to why we, as Black women, are constantly left feeling helpless at the hands of medical providers. We actually have slavery to blame for furthering the medicalization of childbirth and the professionalization of medicine. In 1808, when the Trans-atlantic slave trade ended, slaveholders began to see Black women's reproduction as something they could profit from. Once this happened, they sought out consultation for women's reproduction, which birthed the industry of obstetrics and gynecology on southern plantations, an industry of predominantly white men of course.

As this industry developed, they took a strong look at their competition and dismantled the infrastructure that once served as a woman-centered, safe place. Gradually, minimally trained white male physicians took childbirth, a process meant to be a biological, social, and cultural process, and minimized it down to just a biological process. By interfering with the cultural and social aspects, they transformed pregnancy and childbirth into a series of unfolding events that reflect the choices made by the physicians and their slaveholder clients. Slave women's ideas about what was fitting and effective for their bodies were soon swept away as ignorant folktales.

Unfortunately, since slaves were not respected for their experience or knowledge, doctors and slaves were not able to bridge the gap between holistic and surgical approaches to childbirth, as each judged his or her methods to be superior. Doctors claimed scientific certainty based on reason and knowledge acquired through literacy and professional associations. Enslaved women and early midwives, in contrast, cited their traditions where knowledge was acquired through revelation, a study of the environment, and social relationships. Doctors subsequently joined forces with slaveholders to exercise control over enslaved women's health and medical practices, and the distrust for the medical industry was birthed.

Doctors continued to focus more on identifying diagnoses and establishing cures, which led to the foundation of doctors rarely observing psychosocial circumstances and environmental factors. Doctors tended to view medicine and spirituality as separate fields of study. Black women considered doctors neglectful of practices important for ensuring the well-being of mother and child. They felt women's illnesses should be left in the hands of women, not men. And not much has changed. Like patients today, Black women back then preferred that their birth attendants understood and respected their social circumstances and values, their fears, aspirations, joys, and sorrows. From the very beginning, when doctors intervened, women felt misunderstood and dismissed and were following the agendas of the slaveholders and their professional wishes[1].

If you know anything about the current state of birth in America, you will find that these sentiments are still relevant today. Although some of the stakeholders have changed (hospitals, insurance companies, government), the narrative is still the same - women find their right to birth under strict control, feel unsupported, and find their feelings regularly being dismissed.

DISENFRANCHISEMENT OF MIDWIVES

In West Africa, it was once customary for delivery to occur with the woman squatting on the ground surrounded by sisters and female relatives, some of whom functioned as midwives. America continues to do things differently due to its roots in racism and its competitive nature. The disenfranchisement of Midwives is

---

[1] Birthing a slave: Motherhood and Medicine in the Antebellum South; Marie Jankins Schwartz.

no different. While most wealthy industrialized countries, such as Sweden, Japan, and the United Kingdom still rely heavily on midwives, the US is at 92% of births being attended by OB/GYNs.

During slavery, West African midwives tended to the births of whites and Blacks on southern plantations. After emancipation, African American midwives continued to take care of both black and white poor women in most rural parts of the South, where they were referred to as "granny midwives." While other white women grew accustomed to using the new OB/GYNs established initially for slave reproduction.

Unlike in Europe, where midwifery laws were national, in America, midwifery laws were local and varied widely. With few midwifery schools, laws requiring education couldn't be enforced. And with few doctors positioned or willing to attend to poor women, it wasn't practical to outlaw midwives. Midwives in most states practiced without government control until the 1920s. And even today, the regulation of midwifery varies from state to state.

By the beginning of the 20th century, midwives attended only about half of all births in the U.S., and physicians attended the other half.

A series of events between 1910 and 1920 set the stage for doctors to seize the traditional role of the midwife and laid the foundation for a pathology-oriented medical model of childbirth in this country. Two reports on medical education, published in 1910 and 1912, concluded that America's obstetricians were poorly trained. To improve obstetrics training, one report recommended hospitalization for all deliveries and the gradual abolition of midwifery.

Once midwives were pushed out, it gave way to a more medical and intolerable birth process, and "twilight sleep" was introduced in 1914. Twilight sleep was induced through a combination of morphine for relief of pain, and scopolamine, an amnesiac that caused women to have no memories of giving birth. It became widely accepted as medical progress until later when negative effects were reported. Women were incoherent and a danger to themselves, babies were comatose and pulled out using forceps. It was horrible! The following year, 1915, Dr. Joseph DeLee declared birth a pathological experience that destroys both mother and baby. He disregarded the natural process of birth and laid the foundation for what we today call "the sequence of interventions". He changed the focus of healthcare during labor and delivery from one of responding to problems as they arose, to one where problems were prevented through the routine use of interventions. This change led to medical interventions being applied not just to the relatively small number of women who had a diagnosed problem, but to every woman in labor.

BEWARE OF INTERVENTIONS.

For the average, young, healthy woman, this could easily be your first encounter with inpatient care. Therefore, like me, you might initially be oblivious to what is known as the "Cascade of Inventions." This simply means that using one intervention can lead to the need for more interventions. The problem with this is that although the intervention solves one problem, it then creates new problems that are "solved" with further interventions, which may in turn create even more problems. By altering the natural process of labor, you are inherently opening the door for additional maternity interventions due to unintended effects.

Common maternity choices that lead to a "cascade of interventions" include the following:

- Using medications to induce labor
- Using synthetic oxytocin medicine ("Pitocin") to create more intense contractions
- Epidural to cease sensation below the waist
- Being confined to a bed while in labor

These choices cause additional interventions by interfering with natural hormones that move labor and birth along. Oftentimes, there is no need to rush the birth process. Impatience and anxiety can seep in but give the body and the baby time to prepare. Trust that they will engage when they are ready. By abstaining from intervention, you are also avoiding:

- Creating opportunities for infection
- Having undesirable effects on your baby
- The option to tear due to lack of sensation
- Longer recovery times
- Disconnection
- Troubles breastfeeding

Interventions often leave women feeling as though their bodies have somehow failed them when the sequence of events was triggered by common modern maternity practices. This leads to the development of false narratives around the inability to experience labor happily, naturally, and without extreme pain. Perhaps, more mothers would have positive stories to share if there were fewer unnecessary inductions that lead to subsequent events being outside of their control.

Let me paint you a picture of how Cascade of Interventions works. Take the epidural for example. Epidurals can provide highly effective pain relief during labor, but they also increase the risk of experiencing a sudden drop in blood pressure, longer labor, difficulty moving about, difficulty urinating, difficulty pushing the baby out, fever, and other negative side effects.

Following the epidural, an electronic fetal monitor, IV fluids, and bladder catheter are often used to monitor, prevent, or treat these side effects of the epidural. Eventually, labor is slowed down by the epidural and distractions. Now Pitocin is introduced to try and synthetically speed things up. The baby will encounter some effects from exposure to these medications, leading to a reduced heart rate and drowsiness. The reduced heart rate will often call for an emergency C-section or even cause extreme worry for the mother causing her to disengage from her maternal instincts to work with the baby resulting in a delay in progression. The epidural may have increased the woman's likelihood of developing a fever, which can make doctors worry that the baby has a fever. This leads to blood tests and antibiotics for the baby after birth. Depending on the outcome and length of this process, you and your birthing partner may be exhausted and send your baby to the nursery. This separation can interfere with mother-baby bonding and breastfeeding. The simple choice to have an epidural has now led to an additional 6 or 7 interventions.

DO YOUR RESEARCH

Birth spaces have become one of the most dangerous places for us as Black women. Knowing this, we must arm ourselves with support and knowledge more now than ever before, to create healthy and safe Black birthing spaces. If you find yourself in a position requiring pain relief, it is important to have a complete understanding of their impact and what you are signing up for. It is also important to know what each drug administered, or surgical procedure done, entails and how it will affect your body, your baby, and your birthing outcomes. Remember that epidurals and C-sections are not the only medical interventions available and are often not the first or the last interventions. While it should be the responsibility of your provider to ensure informed consent, we must first hold ourselves accountable for researching the facts before entering these birth spaces. It's highly unlikely that you'll be able to give informed consent while you're in the middle of a 5-hour long period of back-to-back contractions. It's even more highly unlikely if you have never heard of the drug being offered. Don't let this be you.

It's also important to note that everyone's tolerability and reaction to medication looks different. To ensure that you are informed and prepared once you enter your birthing space, here is a list of common medications that might be offered during childbirth:

Pitocin: Pitocin is typically introduced when your contractions stall or when they aren't strong enough to help labor progress. Pitocin acts like the natural hormone your body produces during labor called Oxytocin, which helps start the labor process and helps you push out your baby.

Although Pitocin can speed up your labor, sometimes it can cause intolerable contractions that are too quick or too strong. This often leads to more pressure for an epidural to provide release from manufactured contractions that are unbearable. This can make your baby's heart rate drop. For this reason, your birthing team will closely monitor you and your baby after they give you Pitocin.

Narcotics (also called opioids): These are pain relievers that act on the whole nervous system—not just a specific area—to lessen pain. Narcotics are often given early in labor and can help you relax. They ease dull labor pains but do not block them.

You can have narcotics by an IV line or injection. If you get an IV, you may be able to control your level of relief during labor by pushing a button that releases a fixed amount into your bloodstream. Pain relief begins within minutes, and you can still get an epidural or spinal block (see below) later in labor. The downside to taking narcotics is that it causes drowsiness and can lead to nausea or vomiting. Due to the impairment that they cause, you will not be free to move. This will hinder you from getting into optimal positions for labor progression. Also, if you have narcotics too close to delivery, they can slow your baby's breathing and heartbeat.

Narcotics typically offered during childbirth include meperidine (Demerol®), morphine, fentanyl, butorphanol (Stadol®), and nalbuphine (Nubain®).

Epidurals: Epidurals are the most common type of pain relief used during labor and delivery in the United States, and they can be administered for both vaginal and cesarean births. It allows you to be awake and participate during childbirth while having little to no sensation.

An epidural involves placing a catheter in the lower back, next to the spinal cord. This allows anesthetic medicine to be delivered through the catheter as needed during labor, lessening, or blocking all sensations below the waist. You should notice relief about 10 to 20 minutes after you get an epidural.

However, an epidural can cause your blood pressure to drop, which in turn, can cause the baby's heartbeat to slow. It can also cause low-grade fevers as well as severe headaches if your healthcare provider pierces the covering of the spinal cord while placing the catheter. Some women's labor slows down after an epidural. Epidurals also cause mobility to be hampered during labor, not allowing you to move to aid in labor progression. Women also experience a longer recovery and are unable to walk or hold their baby without assistance.

Spinal Block: This medication is like an epidural in that it lessens or blocks sensation below the waist while allowing you to be awake and alert throughout the birthing process. It also shares some of the same risks and potential side effects. However, a spinal block is a shot of anesthetic into the fluid surrounding the spine. A spinal block provides immediate pain relief but wears off within an hour or two, unlike an epidural. Because of their unique benefits, sometimes a combination of an epidural and spinal block is given during labor for quick as well as continuous relief.

Pudendal Block: This is a numbing medicine your doctor may inject into your vagina and nearby pudendal nerve late in labor, often just before the baby is delivered. The nerve block, which provides some pain relief to the lower part of your vagina and vulva, may also be used if the doctor is calling for an episiotomy (an incision in the tissue between the vaginal opening and anus).

Let me remind you that I did not find birth to be a painful process. There were moments of discomfort, but I would not classify birth as so unbearable that it requires pain relief. I chose to take advantage of comfort measures which I will share below.

Now that you know this, I cannot stress enough the importance of finding a provider who uses interventions only on a case-by-case basis and not as a standard of care. Feel free to rip this page out and take it with you to the hospital for reference if need be. I hope it serves as guidance to help you make more informed decisions and to be aware of the complexity of interventions and the major role that they play in birth outcomes.

As you begin attending your prenatal appointments, take a serious look at how they are making you feel. Are you feeling heard? Do you feel respected? Does this feel like a collaborative effort? Are your feelings validated? Is there any mention of options during your labor? Are you feeling included in decisions? This is one of the most important decisions during the process of ensuring you and your baby are in good hands. Speak up now and do your research. Make it known early that you plan to be the lead on your birthing experience.

Alternatively, there is a broad list of comfort measures that will be typically explored by your doula, and in any birthing preparation classes that you attend. A holistic approach to coping with pain and indeterminate length labor involves the use of the Three Rs: Relaxation, Rhythm, and Ritual. The truth is that some women cope well with discomfort and stress, while others find it downright overwhelming and that's ok. It doesn't make coping holistically impossible; it simply means you should prepare just as you're doing right now. Explore methods and find peace in the process of bringing your beautiful baby earthside. These comfort measures are used to ease birthing discomfort during labor while keeping the birth process progressive and keeping you grounded in your purpose. Welcome these comfort measures to serve as a distraction from the temporary discomfort and pain. This is a time for minimal stimulation and full focus.

Use this list as a guide to find the labor comforts that work for you. Be aware that when you are in active labor, you may prefer more deliberate and rhythmic moves.

- Tension release
- Rhythmic breathing
- Hydrotherapy
- Dim lighting
- Bearing down
- Cold/warm pack
- Counterpressure for hips and back
- Rhythmic movements
- Attention focusing
- Shower/bath
- Double hip squeeze
- Rolling pressure
- Abdominal lifting
- Hands and knees
- Kneeling and leaning over a ball, chair, or couch
- Lunges
- Walking
- Slow dancing
- Hip circles

- Lifting of the belly
- Underarm back support
- Hand and foot massage
- Acupressure
- Hand holding
- Side-lying with a pillow between your legs

In addition to your birth partner or doula supporting you with the physical comfort measures above, your mind will also appreciate the following comfort measures:
Reminders and suggestions

- Encouragement and reassurance
- Compliments
- Undivided attention
- Tracking contractions
- Patience
- Immediate physical support to contractions
- Aid in creating rhythms and relaxation
- Taking charge
- Hugs, kisses, and caresses
- Play affirmations or music

Now that I have shared my experience with choosing a provider, the history behind providers, and the options available for labor management, I'll leave you with a guide to assist you in choosing the provider that best aligns with your ideology, vision, and/or current circumstances. However, please remember that our bodies and stories vary, so to make an informed decision, your story matters. I am only here to encourage you to birth in healthy and safe spaces, ones that resonate with what you genuinely want, desire, and possibly need.

Here are a few questions to consider when choosing between a Midwife or an OB/GYN:

1. Is your pregnancy low risk?
2. Do you want to explore more holistic approaches?
3. Do you want more support or advice on the transition to parenthood?
4. Is vaginal birth a priority for you?
5. Do you have any plans for pain management?
6. Did you previously have a C-section?

If you said yes to at least four (4) of these questions, a midwife could be a good choice for you.

Historically, the disciplines of midwifery and obstetrics are rooted in different pieces of training and origins. Overall, you will find that midwives tend to see more births in their most natural state during training than both physicians and obstetricians. Because of their training, midwives are experts in the process of experiencing birth with little to no interventions and preventing birth complications. While physicians and obstetricians see more complications during their training and become experts in handling birth complications.

The core value of midwives is to affirm the power and strength of women and the importance of their health in the well-being of families, communities, and nations. Their practices allow for prenatal care that reduces stress and anxiety in expectant mothers. Midwives help the progression of labor by encouraging mothers and giving them one-on-one support. OB/GYNs are often not permitted or trained to take the time and space to support what is naturally needed to help labor progression. Midwives also provide holistic approaches to labor-management and culturally sensitive prenatal and postnatal support. While OB/GYNs lean towards interventions and surgical solutions to have quicker turnovers and provide pain management for patients.

Midwives believe in watchful waiting and non-intervention in normal processes, while acknowledging appropriate use of interventions and technology for current or potential health problems. While OB/GYNs are trained to constantly check dilation and perform other monitoring activities, which can easily be labeled as early intervention. Although the midwife practice I birthed with followed the standards of weekly appointments in the final month of pregnancy, there was no rush on my dilation. My dilation check was reserved for when I arrived at the hospital during active labor.

Midwives hold the knowledge of prenatal care as well as how to help mothers in birth spaces. They recognize that women often incur an undue burden of risk when their rights are violated. Unfortunately, many hospitals have opposing agendas and priorities obstructing them from holding space for women to experience labor and delivery freely without undue acceleration and excessive intervention.

Midwives are a great option for low-risk mothers and if you happen to be a high risk, I encourage you to push for combination care. This will ensure that you receive some scope of full support. For instance, if you are interested in having a VBAC, you can work with a midwife who specializes in VBAC. Often in this situation, they will ensure that an OB is available as a resource if this birth experience is not achievable. This will also ensure that you have a better outcome and informed experience.

Once you have a clearer understanding of the birthing experience you envision for yourself, and if you require any additional care, you will have a clearer picture of the ideal care provider for your birthing experience.

Here are some tips for finding the ideal care provider:

1. Reach out to mothers in your community who have had positive birth experiences. These mothers will likely have insight into local care providers and the type of care that was available to them.
2. Beware of using negative stories as your guide. This will make it harder for you to tell if their stories are a result of being cared for at a high interventions hospital, just being an unprepared mother, or due to a special cirumstance.
3. Speak with a Doula. Doulas have experience helping many mothers at local birth centers and hospitals, they are a wealth of knowledge regarding the hospital dynamics surrounding birth and can steer you in a positive direction to meet your birthing desires.
4. Create a list of questions to ask your provider. Unfortunately, birth scenarios are often not discussed before implementing them. This pattern is causing trauma and should be considered as a lack of informed consent. I encourage you to ask your care providers questions regarding induction

methods, what leads them to call for a C-section, Pitocin levels, birth positions, and anything else you discover on this journey that you want to unpack.

To help you get started, here are some questions to ask any potential care providers:

a. In your opinion, how can a mother prepare to give birth free of interventions? (You want a provider who believes that what women do leading up to and during labor has an impact.)
b. Do you have any children? Can you tell me about your birth experience? (This is a chance to hear about their thoughts on birth. Listen to hear if their thoughts lean towards dependence on interventions or a belief in a mother's ability.)
c. Can you tell me about a beautiful birth you attended to? (You want to hear about births that inspired your care provider and gives you a valuable gem to take with you on your journey. If you find the care provider is struggling to retrieve an answer, this provider must not see many connected births and is implementing the cascade of interventions too often to see the beauty in birth.)
d. How are you making sure that Black mothers feel safe in birth spaces? (Trust your gut here. You are the Black mother, and how this provider makes you feel matters!)
e. What are your thoughts on a mother going past her estimated due date? (You want a provider who believes that

your estimated due date is indeed just that - an estimated due date. Ultimately, it is the baby who decides when to arrive and you want a care provider who respects your right to wait an additional 7-10 days if neither of you is at any risk.)

As you take control of your birthing experience by asking questions, be aware that many doctors and midwives are also affected by our harmful birthing system and may be viewing birth through a jaded lens. Care providers that often intervene may feel attacked and defensive about your questions. This is not the right provider for someone like you who is looking to be engaged in your birthing experience. You want someone who finds joy in supporting the birthing mother and is more than happy to ensure that you feel safe and can trust them.

The next chapter is designed to equip you with the tools you need to put together your birthing team. It is also where you will find a "Birth Plan Template". Take the time to prepare for your baby's birth with your team. Go through this list together and establish a plan of action for the big day!

In the meantime, here are some additional questions to ask possible care providers:

- What is your philosophy around birth?
- How long have you been practicing, and how many births have you attended as the primary attendant?
- Do you practice alone or with others? If with others, what is their experience? Do they share your beliefs and manner of practice?

- Who attends births for you when you are away?
- Where do you attend births, and can I take a tour?
- How can I reach you?
- How often will I see you during these next months?
- What kind of birth preparation do you recommend?
- What tests do you recommend for pregnant women? Why?
- How do you define and handle complications?
- Do you provide labor support and stay with women throughout labor? If not, do the nurses provide one-on-one care for women during labor?
- How do you feel about doulas, labor assistants, or family and friends being present?
- Do you support moving around during labor, changing positions, and eating and drinking?
- Will I see you after the birth takes place?
- If I want to hold my baby right after birth, breastfeed, and not be separated, will that be supported?
- Under what circumstances do you recommend IVs, continuous electronic fetal monitoring, Pitocin, episiotomy, forceps or vacuum, cesarean section, or immediate clamping of the baby's umbilical cord? What is your cesarean rate? Episiotomy rate? Induction rate?
- What is your protocol for the birth of twins and breech births?
- Do you attend vaginal births after cesareans (VBACs)?

5

ASSEMBLE THE REST OF YOUR BIRTHING TEAM

Once you have chosen your provider, it's time to assemble the rest of your birth team. You want to cultivate a team that will provide you with the wisdom, and emotional and physical support you need to bring your baby earth-side. This team should work with you to ensure that your wishes are met, they must also remind you of your vision for birth and assist you with any challenging moments that might arise. The best way to fill that void is by adding an experienced doula to your team. A doula should not be confused with a midwife or OB/GYN. A doula is a non-medical birth support person, and they are there to support you by providing physical, emotional, and even spiritual support while sharing their knowledge acquired from their own births, other births they have attended, and experience in various medical settings. This gives them the capacity to support you in a way that your mother, auntie, husband, or partner simply cannot. Doulas have studied the art of birth and how to make birth a more comfortable experience. Their role is to provide consistent birth support to the mother and family, no matter what decisions the mother makes or how she chooses to give birth. The presence of another person, in which human-to-human interaction with caring behaviors is practiced, is proven to be therapeutic,

The word doula is derived from the Greek word known as women's servant. Women have always served other women through life experiences, and childbirth is no different. When women support women in birth spaces it makes way for more positive outcomes and more informed decisions. With a doula's support, women are less likely to have pain-relief medications administered and are less likely to have a cesarean birth. Many women have reported having a more positive childbirth experience with a doula present during their birthing experience. Studies have shown that having a doula as a member of one's birth team decreases the overall cesarean rate by 50%, the length of labor by 25%, the use of Pitocin by 40%, and requests for an epidural by 60%[2].

While doulas are not formally trained in obstetrics, they are trained and experienced in supporting women through prenatal preparation, childbirth, and postpartum care. This means that they plan to be with you every step of the way. They take the time to build a strong rapport with you and your family, allowing them to provide customized support. Commonly providing couples with one-on-one birth education and comfort measures practice. Their focus is on continuous support in all disciplines

---

2   Americanpregnancy.org; What is a Doula.

and advocacy to a mother who is expecting, is experiencing birth, and postpartum. This exceeds the capacity of other health professionals such as doctors, nurses, and some midwives, who have other patients and obligations during and right after their patients' births. It is indeed common to enter your birthing space in a hospital with a complete group of strangers ready to assist in the delivery of your baby. This is very much the opposite of how births were once inherently done. Doulas help fill this void by being someone you have built a relationship with, that you can rely on to be there the entire time, while also being knowledgeable about hospitals and birth centers. Doctors, midwives, and nurses are interchangeable, but your doula is committed to only you! Note that the doula's role and agenda are tied solely to your agenda. You are their primary responsibility. They do not report to a hospital administrator, nurse, midwife, or doctor, they report to you. Although doulas are not associated with the US medical system, they have experienced how that system works and doesn't work for its birthing mothers. As a result, they can support you at home before you even enter the birthing center or hospital. This allows them to have an accurate story of your birth process and assist you in decisions regarding your progression and timelines if need be. I have outlined some specific ways below that doulas provide support during the birth experience. Please use this information to guide you with establishing preferences when interviewing and having preparation meetings with your doula.

    The physical support provided by doulas allows the laboring mother to maintain a sense of control, comfort, and confidence.

Doulas often use the power of touch and massage to reduce stress and anxiety during labor. According to physicians, Marshal Klaus and John Kennel, massage helps stimulate the production of natural oxytocin. The pituitary gland secretes natural oxytocin to the bloodstream (causing uterine contractions) and to the brain (resulting in feelings of well-being and drowsiness, along with a higher pain threshold.

Here are some examples of how a doula may support you physically.

- Soothing with touch using massage, counter pressure, or a rebozo
- Helping to create a calm environment, like dimming lights and arranging curtains.
- Suggesting and preparing hydrotherapy
- Assisting with relieving any fluids or waste from the body
- Providing food or liquid nourishment to keep you hydrated and fueled.

Doulas engage laboring mothers with emotional support to ensure that they feel cared for and feel a sense of pride and empowerment before and after giving birth. Since birth can be unpredictable and go through various stages, doulas are intentional about enhancing the mother's ability to have positive birth memories regarding the birth experience. They're often able to help work through any fear or self-doubt that can occur during intense labor. Additionally, they can work with the mother to debrief, process their birth experience, and celebrate.

The grounding that a doula provides allows for women to make more informed decisions and takes some of the surprises out of the birth experience.

One of my favorite perks to having a doula is that they provide informational support by keeping the mother and her partner informed about what's going on throughout labor. They also provide them with access to evidence-based information about birthing options. This can take so many forms, from preparation for birth to postpartum care. Doulas have often gone through this process many times that they are such a wealth of knowledge and resources. They work with many partners and can help engage your partner in the process, giving them the tools that they need to help you feel supported throughout labor.

The most skilled and confident doulas have mastered advocacy. Advocacy can take many forms in the birthing room. Local doulas may be familiar with hospital staff and interventions that are often enforced at certain hospitals. Doulas can assist in creating space for you to make informed decisions, away from medical professionals, that align with your birth plan and previously established vision. Some examples of advocacy that doulas have described include:

- Encouraging the mother or their partner to ask questions and verbalize their preferences.
- Asking the mother what she wants
- Supporting the mother's decision
- Amplifying the mother's voice if she is being dismissed, ignored, or not being heard.

- Creating space and time for the birthing family so that they can ask questions, gather evidence-based information, and make decisions without feeling pressured.
- Facilitating communication between the parents and their care providers
- Teaching the mother and partner positive communication techniques
- If a mother is not aware that a provider is about to perform an intervention, the doula can point out what it appears the nurse or physician is about to do and ask the birthing person if they have any questions about what is about to happen.

Remember that the presence of a doula can be beneficial no matter what type of birth you are planning or will experience. A doula's skilled support will make way for fewer interventions and embracing holistic practices and rituals. The primary goal is to have a safe, pleasant, and connected experience.

For women who have decided to have a medicated birth, your doula will still provide emotional, informational, and physical support through labor and the administration of medications. Doulas work alongside medicated mothers to help them deal with potential side effects. Doulas may also help with other needs where medication may be inadequate because even with medication, there is likely to be some degree of discomfort.

For mothers not expecting or expecting to have a cesarean, a doula can help provide constant support and encouragement. Cesarean sections can often result in a mother experiencing many emotions of loneliness or disconnection from the process or the baby. A doula can be of service to those emotions and the C-section process. This can free your partner up to attend to the baby and accompany the newborn to the nursery if there are complications.

Our doula, Fatima Abdallah, was such an essential part of our birthing experience. In our first interview with her, both my partner and I initially took to her calm but assertive spirit. As a mother of four, I felt confident that she had the hands-on experience that I was looking for as a new mother. Once we hired her, she quickly set up a continuous line of communication and scheduled our in-person meetings. These in-person meetings served as additional birth education for us since we took advantage of birthing classes associated with the midwife center. She facilitated mock labor practices, provided resources including a subscription for Hypnobirthing and postpartum books, and helped us lay out our birth preferences. This included how to make decisions regarding interventions and initial newborn care. She also took the time to help us explore the most optimal environment for laboring and key elements that could keep me grounded whether at home or in the hospital. I was able to identify smells, lighting, and other comfort measures that enhanced my birth experience.

My partner was not left out, she equipped him with techniques to use for comfort measures, pain management, and fetal positioning. This gave both of us the confidence we needed to labor at home for as long as possible as a family. We labored alone for almost 8 hours before our doula joined us to provide

> You should not go into labor and delivery blind to the process or the distress signals, because when you and your birth tribe are not knowledgeable, you forfeit your power to stand up for your family in a labor and delivery room.

relief to my partner and additional support for me. Whoever your birthing team is, make sure that they know the labor process too. Whether it's your girlfriend, sibling, mother, husband, someone will need to know the difference between early and active labor, how to track contractions and when to make the call to your birth location when time gets tight!

My partner played an active role in my labor and delivery. He was present and engaging in classes, this allowed him to successfully manage our day in labor. We planned to labor at home for as long as possible, so we created an elaborate list of things to do as we prepared ourselves for the marathon. As I look back on Mother's Day weekend 2019, I may have started labor earlier than I initially thought. New mothers are often told that labor is much longer the first time and that they may experience false labor, so I took that message and refused to get my hopes up too easily. The day my labor began, we went to an open house, I cooked dinner and we watched Netflix, all while in early labor. JB, my fiancé at the time, was paying close attention as it appeared my labor had become intensified. He began to track my contractions, or, as we referred to them at the time, birth waves. He ran me a warm bath as planned and set a peaceful tone in the bathroom of our 1-bedroom apartment. Dim lights and our birthing playlist. He continued to track my birth waves and apply pressure to my body as the waves came. While simultaneously contacting our doula and the hospital for additional support and preparation. He was strong and intentional as he drove us to the hospital and gave minute-by-minute updates as we cautiously maneuvered through the early morning streets of the district. For this, I am forever grateful. His actions gave me the space I needed to solely focus on breathing our baby down the canal. I was able to rest in between birth waves and able to connect with our baby on a higher level without an ounce of anxiety or distractions. This focus is essential. This is not the time for unnecessary conversations, scrolling, or contacting anyone. As I intentionally shut the rest of the world out, I solely listened to my body and baby for directions.

    I hear so many women say they were too tired to attend birthing classes, but I urge you to attend for the knowledge and the power! You will learn the stages of labor, the female anatomy, and physiology, imperative information that will allow you to make informed decisions for your baby, and if medical assistance is indeed necessary. You should not embark on labor and delivery blind to the process or the distress signals, because when you and your birth tribe are not knowledgeable, you forfeit your power to stand up for your family in a labor and delivery room. Doctors, midwives, and other medical professionals are only there to guide you throughout your birthing experience. You are ultimately responsible for your outcomes and decisions. Be an active participant in your birth experience because you will be reminded of this day every day in your baby's eyes.

By taking this crucial step in preparation, you will be empowered to do things you didn't know you were capable of. This strength has an impact on you and your baby's outcomes. To help you get started with claiming your power of choice and to bring you a step closer to being able to advocate for yourself, your baby, and your family, I have put together some resources at the end of this chapter to guide you on your path to experiencing a calm, knowledgeable, well-informed, well-prepared birthing process. Resources include a birth plan that will help you put your birthing ideals on paper; a chapter checklist; and a list of questions to ask your doula during the initial meeting and throughout the process. I hope you find these resources useful and helpful.

The power of the birth plan isn't the actual plan itself. It's the process of becoming informed about all your options. Use this as a roadmap to get informed about interventions and how to prepare for the birth you envision. Although birth can be unpredictable, if you go into birth with an understanding of your options, you are more likely to make decisions with confidence. An inclusive birth plan prepares you, teaches you, and will help minimize the likelihood of birth trauma.

HOW TO AVOID A C-SECTION:

In the previous chapters, I discussed how medical interventions often lead to C-sections and more complicated births. Now, I want to share a list of things to do to avoid a C-section. These tips should be considered when building your birth plan.

1. Avoid induction. If your care provider suggests an induction, inquire about the reasoning and request additional time. For example, if it's Friday, request to return after the weekend. This will give you time to try some natural ways to induce, you will find a few tips on how to naturally induce birth in the next chapter undernutrition. Inductions can work for some moms, usually, moms who have birthed before. But typically, a first-time mom will not have much luck with an induction.
2. Avoid an epidural. Epidurals reduce sensation and mobility. This will slow down labor and increase your likelihood of being diagnosed as 'failure to progress'.
3. Stay home for as long as possible or plan a home birth. Look out for telltale signs to require medical support, such as water breaking or any fluid that is not blood or clear.

25 QUESTIONS TO ASK YOUR POTENTIAL DOULA

1. What type of training do you have?
2. How long have you practiced as a doula?
3. How many births have you attended?
4. What's your philosophy around birth?
5. Why did you become a doula?
6. How would you describe your style as a doula?

7. How do you prepare partners for labor?
8. How do you most often support women during labor?
9. Do you provide postpartum services?
10. Do you have a backup doula?
11. How many clients do you take in a month?
12. Have you given birth? Did you have a doula? Describe your birth experience.
13. Are you familiar with my birth location? If so, what was your experience like?
14. How many visits do you include for prenatal and postpartum care?
15. May I text, call and email you questions?
16. Have you attended home births?
17. Have you attended births that resulted in a C-section? If so, how did you continue to provide support?
18. How do you work with doctors and midwives?
19. At what point during labor will you join us? How long can you stay?
20. What coping techniques do you find the most helpful?
21. How do you feel about epidurals? Other pain medications? Pitocin?
22. How long do you stay with the mother after birth?
23. Do you have experience with breastfeeding instructions?
24. Do you offer any additional services?
25. What are your fees and packages?

BIRTH PLAN CHECKLIST

My Name: _____

Labor Companions: _____

Healthcare Provider: _____

LABOR PREFERENCES

- [ ] Dim Lighting
- [ ] Quiet
- [ ] Play Music
- [ ] Wear my own clothing.
- [ ] Bring things in from home, like blankets or photos.
- [ ] Aromatherapy scents
- [ ] Video/photos taken by_____

MOBILITY

- [ ] I prefer to maintain all mobility, including walking and changing positions.
- [ ] I prefer to be able to move around in bed only and get up to use the bathroom.

☐ Mobility is not important to me, and I understand that if I get an epidural, I may be confined to bed and need a urinary catheter to go to the bathroom.

HYDRATION AND NOURISHMENT

☐ I would like to eat light snacks and drink clear fluids whenever possible during labor.
☐ It would not bother me to have an IV for hydration if necessary.
☐ I prefer a saline lock if the placement of an IV is required by my hospital, but no fluids or medication are needed during my labor.

MONITORING

☐ I prefer my baby to be monitored as minimally as possible.
☐ I would like as much monitoring as possible.
☐ I prefer a method that allows me to remain mobile.
☐ Fetal monitoring in bed is fine with me.

PAIN RELIEF

☐ I prefer to lean on comfort measures.
☐ I prefer that pain medication not be offered to me.
☐ I prefer to use medication as the last possible option.
☐ Pitocin
☐ Narcotics

☐ Spinal Block
☐ Epidural

AUGMENTATION METHODS TO SPEED UP LABOR IF MY LABOR SLOWS DOWN,

I would:

☐ Like to try nonmedical methods like walking and using upright labor positions.
☐ Prefer that my bag of water breaks on its own.
☐ Prefer that my practitioner breaks my water.
☐ Prefer to receive an IV of Pitocin only after all other methods are tried, and only if medically necessary.
☐ Not mind having an IV of Pitocin and understand the benefits and risks involved.

PUSHING

☐ I prefer to wait to push until I feel the urge or until my baby descends.
☐ I would like to use a variety of positions during pushing.
☐ I would like a mirror placed at the foot of the bed so I can watch my baby's birth.
☐ I would like to push whenever I feel like it.
☐ I would like to be directed as to when to push.
☐ I prefer any natural tearing over an episiotomy.
☐ I would like to avoid forceps and/or vacuum extraction unless necessary.

- [ ] I would like to touch my baby's head as it crowns.
- [ ] I would like my healthcare provider to hand me the baby immediately if there aren't any complications.

BIRTH AND BABY CARE

- [ ] I would like to hold my baby for skin-to-skin contact immediately after birth.
- [ ] I would like to breastfeed as soon as possible.
- [ ] I would like _____ to cut the umbilical cord.
- [ ] I would like to wait to have the cord cut until the baby receives all the blood from the placenta.
- [ ] I would like to donate the umbilical cord blood.
- [ ] I would like to keep the umbilical cord.
- [ ] I would like to keep the placenta.
- [ ] I would prefer that routine hospital procedures be done while I hold my baby.
- [ ] I would like all routine tests, shots, and procedures for my newborn.
- [ ] I prefer to choose the tests and shots that are done.
- [ ] I am breastfeeding exclusively and don't want my baby to be given pacifiers, bottles, or formula.
- [ ] I do not wish to send my baby to the nursery.
- [ ] If I have a boy, I prefer to have him circumcised.
- [ ] I do not want my baby boy to be circumcised.
- [ ] I would like my baby's hearing to be tested.

IN CASE OF A CESAREAN

- [ ] I would like _____ to accompany me during surgery.
- [ ] If possible, I would like two people to accompany me.
- [ ] If anesthesia is a choice for me, I would prefer an epidural.
- [ ] If anesthesia is a choice for me, I would prefer a spinal block.
- [ ] If possible, I would like music played in the operating room.
- [ ] I would like the drape/screen lowered during surgery so I can see the birth.
- [ ] I would like the surgeon to describe the surgery as he or she goes along.
- [ ] I would like to have videos or photos taken.
- [ ] I would like my support person to cut the cord.
- [ ] I would like my support person to do skin to skin with the baby.
- [ ] I would like to have at least one arm released so I can hold my baby right away.
- [ ] I would like to breastfeed as soon as possible in the recovery room.

8

PREPARING YOUR BODY AND BELLY FOR DELIVERY

Prenatal activity has always been rooted in necessity, race, cultural ideals, and social status. As far back as in Biblical times, it was observed that Hebrew slave women had an easier time giving birth than their sedentary Egyptian mistresses. Spartan women BC were encouraged to harden their bodies with exercise to decrease the pain of childbearing.

Our expecting ancestors were alongside their husbands in cotton fields or serving in plantation homes caring for their owner's wives and children. Sadly, pregnancy was not often a reason to reduce one's workload. And while some of the strenuous activity imposed on slaves led to miscarriages, many of the women were in optimal physical strength to birth in cotton fields or at their quarters accompanied by their resident midwife. Some circumstances did call for bedrest just like it does today, however, most women remained active, and this was a good thing.

From conception to postpartum recovery, a body undergoes extensive changes with frequently evolving adaptations. Physical and hormonal changes occur gradually throughout 9 months of pregnancy, and these are reversed in a matter of weeks during postpartum recovery. Skeletal tissue, muscle and connective fibers, blood volume, cardiac output, body weight, and posture are all affected. Your body will greatly benefit from a well-established physical activity and nutritional plan if you don't already have one in place.

The current stationary lifestyle tied to American culture and technology does not innately prepare our bodies for pregnancy or birthing. After the first 3 months, you will typically gain 1 pound a week and will be carrying 6-10 pounds of baby weight once you reach full term until the birthing experience is complete. Then you will spend anywhere from 12-24 hours in labor, this can be shorter or longer. Labor will test your physical and mental stamina.

You can prepare yourself for positive outcomes by getting your body into optimal shape for birthing. Birth will require established endurance and a sprint at the end. And just when you feel you've done all you can do, there will be that final push at the finish line.

Take Jodie Turner-Smith for example, a black actress who opted for a home birth due to the negative birth outcomes associated with Black women and the US medical system. In her British Vogue essay, she shares that her home birth experience lasted four days. On the morning of the third day, she felt as though she was losing resolve. Then she, her partner and their unborn baby shared a moment, and they came together as a family to stay the course. Jodie says she took the time to speak to her baby. Keep in mind that during pregnancy, Jodie was preparing for an action film that involved intense physical activity. Remember, that time is not our enemy and physical conditioning is our best friend.

When it comes to labor, the process is broken down into 3 stages. There is early labor and active labor, the birth of your baby, and birthing the placenta.

STAGE 1: EARLY LABOR AND ACTIVE LABOR

The first stage of labor occurs when you begin to feel regular contractions which cause the cervix to open (dilate) and soften, shorten, and thin (effacement). This allows your baby to move into the birth canal. The first stage is the longest of the three stages. It's divided into two phases of its own — early labor and active labor.

Early labor can be very unpredictable, anywhere from hours to days, but you will know you are experiencing it when you lose your mucus plug. Contractions are typically mild at this point, but your body is working, and you will feel your muscles tightening and releasing. You should keep moving, go for a walk, bounce on your birthing ball, go to dinner or prepare your last meal before your new status change.

Active labor is where the real work happens. Your body experiences more intense contractions and your cervix will actively dilate from 6cm to 9cm. These contractions should be consistent, stronger, and grow closer and closer together. It means that your body is working, so do your best to keep your strength by helping your body along. This is where the comfort measures mentioned in the last chapter come into play. This is the time for hip circles on all fours, counter pressure by your doula or partner, and anything that provides rhythm, ritual, and relaxation. This is the time to avoid all distractions and focus on your instinctual nature. This can last for four to eight hours. It is very normal during this time to experience nausea, leg cramps, or an urge to use the bathroom. At this time, you should head to your birthing space or have your midwife present.

STAGE 2: THE BIRTH OF YOUR BABY

It is time to meet your baby! This is known as a transition, the shortest yet most intense moment. If you have made it this far without interventions, you may be able to experience the art of fetal ejection reflex. With trust and security, your body will step into final action, you may feel the need to stand up, get on all fours, squat...with synchronization your baby may naturally expel with a little pushing. Either way, the final process of birth can take anywhere from 15 minutes or up to 2 hours. The key is to push or bear down in sync with each contraction to shorten this period. You should note that epidurals will increase the time it takes to push due to lack of sensation. Since you are unable to feel the contractions, it will decrease the likelihood for you to push when they happen.

If you happen to deliver your baby by C-section, it is still especially important for your recovery that you are in good physical condition. Your body will be in serious repair mode and will need all the strength to repair sutured muscles. Not only that, but you will also have a beautiful new baby that needs your protection from this big new world.

STAGE 3: BIRTHING THE PLACENTA

As you stare in awe at your new miracle of life and enjoy the golden hour of bonding with this beautiful creation, using skin-to-skin contact, you will need to birth the placenta. This may seem a bit daunting after all that you have just accomplished. The placenta is typically birthed about 5-20 minutes after the baby. The hospital procedure is often to push on the stomach and give Pitocin to assist with the birth of the placenta. This is your choice too. You can continue to decline intervention and birth your placenta when your body is ready. Latching the baby can assist with necessary contractions to release the placenta as well. You can also opt to keep your baby attached to the placenta for continuous nutrients for an extended period or often referred to as lotus birth.

Now that you have a better understanding of what you are preparing for, let's talk about the significance and benefits of physical activity during pregnancy and birth. Staying active is essential to your preparation for birth. Our physical activity level, as women, usually lies somewhere on a spectrum of highly active to not active at all, the goal is to find a balance and to keep your weight gain at a healthy and manageable level for your body frame. Carrying a growing human being for 9 months will require the use of different muscles, pressure on ligaments, and a robust circulation system, and although you have now come to realize that birth is more than a physical experience, you will want to feel connected to your body. This trust is built through knowing your body's capabilities and nurturing your self-confidence. The body that you build during pregnancy will carry you through postpartum and assist with your recovery process.

It is currently advised that pregnant women get at least 150 minutes a week of moderate exercise, roughly 30 minutes, 5 times a day. Gentle activity is encouraged, such as walking, swimming, or prenatal yoga. If you are already a physically active person, the key is for you to get more out of less and to embrace more restorative activity. Interventions are greatly reduced by this steady flow of activity, and regular exercisers are 75 percent less likely to encounter a forceps delivery, while 55 percent are less likely to have an episiotomy and up to four times less likely to have a Cesarean section. A study found that among well-conditioned women who delivered vaginally, those who had continued training throughout their pregnancy experienced active labor for 4 hours and 24 minutes compared with 6 hours and 22 minutes for those who quit exercise early on.

Simply put, continued physical activity throughout pregnancy will increase the chances of everything listed below:

- Healthy weight gain
- To ease labor and delivery
- To lower your risk of gestational diabetes and hypertension
- Better moods
- To reduce constipation
- To reduce your risk of interventions
- Shorter labor

- Less leg swelling.
- Increase confidence.

I gained a total of 35 pounds during my first pregnancy. On average, women gain anywhere from 25-40 pounds during pregnancy. When I became pregnant, I was lifting weights 3-4 times a week and attending spin and barre classes 2-3 times a week. I continued to follow my active lifestyle upon finding out that I was pregnant while also establishing some healthy boundaries to ensure that I did not overexert myself.

During the first few months, you may feel a little drained and bogged down by nausea associated with hormone shifts as your body prepares itself. However, anticipate your energy to pick up once you hit the second trimester. During the first trimester, I found myself ending my workday with a nap instead of heading straight to the gym. Although this required some adjustment, I found peace in listening to my body.

Here is an overview of my physical activity trimester by trimester. I hope it serves as a useful guide to you on your journey. You will notice that over time, my physical activity gradually decreased, and I became more focused on birth preparation.

Before becoming pregnant, and during my first trimester, my workouts included:

i. High-intensity fitness classes 1-2 days a week
ii. Cardio focused at least 3-4 days a week on a 60-minute spin class or 30-minute elliptical, weight training, and Barre classes

iii. Waking and using public transit

Second trimester:

i. Cardio focused at least 3-4 days a week on a 60-minute spin class or 30-minute elliptical, weight training, and Barre classes
ii. Walking and using public transit

During my third trimester, I started to tone back on my moderate activity and focused on more intentional activity to prepare specifically for labor. To do this, I did the following:

i. Attended prenatal yoga weekly
ii. Attended Barre classes 2-3 times a week
iii. Watched YouTube Fit pregnancy channels
iv. Sat on the birthing ball often
v. Walking and using public transit for prenatal appointments

You may notice extreme fatigue in the first trimester that will return in the third trimester, so be gentle with yourself, every day will certainly be unique. To stay active, I attended Yoga and barre classes right until my due date. I even worked out the night before I went into labor. Remember though, working out at 9 months pregnant can simply mean walking the incline on a treadmill and doing some hip-opening squats for 15 minutes. You do not have to overdo it.

I found Barre and prenatal yoga to be ideal low-impact physical activities for preparing my body for labor. They are both centered around the Goddess Pose. The Goddess Pose is great for opening your hips, while also strengthening your legs. Doing this pose daily can make labor easier because it keeps you open and holding it for minutes at a time prepares your body for being in this position during labor. This heavy emphasis on squats, controlled breathing, and hip opening exercises are key components in labor preparation. Some of the earliest records of birthing show women adopting a sitting, squatting or standing position while in labor. An ancient sculpture from Egypt shows Cleopatra (69 - 30BC) kneeling to give birth, surrounded by five attendants. Evidence of birthing stools and chairs date back to Babylonian times, and surveys conducted in 1882 and 1961 have shown that lying down has never been the norm in traditional cultures[3].

Barre allows you to target the muscle groups that are key to supporting your growing bump. This is to lengthen and strengthen your muscles, which include your glutes, inner thighs, hamstrings, abdominals, pelvic floor, and upper and lower back. When you do this, not only are you staying in optimal shape and managing your pregnancy weight, but you are also making room for your growing baby. This will help you to combat the pain and discomfort often associated with pregnancy. Ultimately, staying strong allows you to feel confident throughout. Remember the day of labor will require strength from your whole body and more specifically your core.

---

[3] As found in https://www.nowtolove.com.au/parenting/pregnancy-birth/lying-down-birth-history-45385

One surprising way to prepare for the endurance test of active labor is through cycling or spin class. This is because cycling incorporates spirit interval training. These intervals require you to push your body to fatigue by pushing your heart, lungs, and muscles a bit further each time. In the middle of an interval, you may feel like you have nothing left to give, but the key is to fight through that feeling to the end of the interval. If you do so, you will find relief, much like birth contractions. Birth contractions will be in intervals, they will start slowly and gradually increase in intensity, but once they reach their peak they will slowly decrease and then you will find relief. Likewise, during labor, as you get closer to transition time, the contractions will become closer together. The rule for wanting to birth without interventions is to head to the hospital when contractions near 3-1-1, which means your contractions are happening every 3 minutes, lasting for 1 full minute, and have been that way for 1 hour. Cycling is a great way to train your mind and body for birth because it creates a pattern of trust in your body.

Another practice that will support your day of labor and recovery is Kegels. They are a must to develop the deep core strength necessary for labor and pushing out your baby. Kegel exercises focus on the muscles that support your bladder, bowels, and uterus. Kegels will assist in a speedy recovery after delivery, including increasing your urinary control. I noticed bladder control deficiency during the first 4 months of postpartum and that was it! It is possible to do permanent damage, so add those Kegels in with your squats or at least while binge-watching Netflix.

Also, feel free to attend your traditional yoga class if you are already a yogi, but forgo the inversions. Incorporating a prenatal yoga class for more intentional breathwork, hip-opening poses, and finding other new mommas is a must. And no hot yoga mommy, until that baby is out! We must not overheat during pregnancy.

The benefits of prenatal yoga include:

- Improved sleep
- Reduced stress
- Increased strength, flexibility, and endurance
- Decreased lower back pain
- Decreased nausea
- Decreased carpal tunnel syndrome
- Decreased headaches
- Reduced risk of preterm labor
- Lowered risk of intrauterine growth restriction (a condition that slows the baby's growth)

Disclaimer: The rule of thumb is, if you were active before becoming pregnant, then continue with the same level of activity as you had before. If you were not active before becoming pregnant, then proceed with caution and consult with your birth professional.

I began experiencing early labor about 1-2 days before active labor. It started with some belly tightening but there was no pain associated with these sensations, just a bit of discomfort. I even continued with my normal activities. I visited friends, did a very low-impact workout that included walking, stretching, and squats, and visited a few open houses. I strongly advise you not to focus that much attention on how much time has passed during early labor but instead allow labor to run its course and give your baby space and time. On the final day, we initiated active labor the same way that we conceived. Shortly afterward, I lost my mucus plug and started to feel more intense contractions. Following an intimate session, a woman's body initiates many functions to propel labor forward, you have contractions from the orgasm, oxytocin from stimulation, and prostaglandins to thin and dilate the cervix. Sex is one of the most natural ways to induce labor. You will find that many medications used to induce labor are manufactured hormones associated with sex.

It became obvious to my partner that I was in active labor, even though I was a bit in denial, still shuffling around the kitchen preparing dinner.

You will find your physical preparation checklist at the end of this chapter. By maintaining a well-regulated, nonstrenuous exercise program initiated in the fourth month or sustained from pre-pregnancy through the postpartum period, you will ensure that you can maintain good physical condition, increase your comfort in pregnancy, deliberately prepare for postpartum recovery, and sustain the necessary muscular activity for the work of childbirth. This will also support your feelings of well-being and confidence that result from regular, whole-body exercise that will enable you to approach childbirth with positive expectations.

Here are a few tips to help you safely stay active while pregnant.

- Monitor your heart rate closely. Remember to take your time and don't try to keep up in fitness classes
- Permit yourself to make modifications
- Do safe abdominal exercises
- Listen to your body and rest when need be
- Engage in less intense workouts in your last 60 days of pregnancy
- Drink a lot of water
- Do Kegels

NUTRIENTS

The high rates of preeclampsia, gestational hypertension, and diabetes associated with Black women are linked to a variety of risk factors while some are linked to irreversible damage from racism and societal pressures that we can't control. Our nutritional choices are not only important to the health of the baby but are also reflected in our energy levels and our ability to have a lowkey pregnancy and delivery. What we consume is something we do have the power to control. Poor health choices can cause or increase our possibilities of being diagnosed with birth complications and can also lead to interventions.

During pregnancy, you'll find that your body needs and craves more nutrients, vitamins, and minerals than you would normally consume. If you're not flooding your body with the proper nutrients, your baby will still take what it needs and leave you a weak, nauseous, and fatigued mama. There is no need to eat for 2 or to double your calories. The rule of thumb is an additional 300 calories a day starting in the second trimester and up to 500 in the final weeks. This may vary by the day. I did not find this necessary every day but there were indeed days when I ate more than others. So, it's important to maintain a more balanced diet for your baby's development and to reduce the chances of mommy being diagnosed with gestational anything. But what does a balanced diet look like?

You are the primary source for everything your baby needs. Your baby will pull all the vitamins and minerals you have consumed, whether you can spare them or not. So, both of you must be getting an adequate amount of nutrition. This is best done by a combination of food and a good natural prenatal vitamin, preferably a food-based one. Here is what should be noted as essential nutrients for Mama and Baby[4].

- Vitamin A – Supports eye, brain, heart, and respiratory development
- Vitamin B6 – Helps red blood cell formation and eases morning sickness
- Vitamin B12 – May prevent neural tube defects and support the placenta
- Choline – Assists in brain formation, liver function, and healthy metabolism

---

4 Book: The Mama Natural by Genevieve Howland.

- Vitamin C – Nourishes the amniotic sac and placenta, good for gum health.
- Vitamin D – Helps mom utilize calcium and strengthens baby's bones
- DHA – Builds baby's brain and promotes a healthy fetal weight
- Vitamin K – Supports your bone formation and healthy blood clotting
- Calcium – Aids bone and teeth development as well as muscle function
- Iron – Helps prevent anemia, low birth weight, and premature delivery
- Iodine – Enhances immune system and healthy thyroid function
- Magnesium – Helps with good blood pressure and blood sugar levels
- Zinc – Supports immune system functions and enzyme functions

Your food selection should be full of the nutrients above to provide energy and support good health for you and your baby. Here's a quick guide to ensure you're reaching all impactful corners of a balanced diet.

- Dark leafy greens – Kale, collard greens, Brussel sprouts, spinach
- Fresh vegetables – Broccoli, cauliflower, bell peppers, and zucchini

- Bright berries – Blueberries, strawberries, pomegranate
- Colorful Fruits – Apples, grapes, mangos, bananas, and pineapples
- High-quality proteins – grass-fed beef, chicken, seafood, eggs, and seeds
- Healthy fats – Yogurt, organic butter, avocado, coconut, and olive oils
- Good Carbs – Sweet potatoes, Red and blue potatoes, carrots, Yams, and plantains
- Whole Grains – Oats, quinoa, buckwheat, and millet

The human body is remarkable and intuitive. A little trust and listening to your body can go a long way. I battled with lactose intolerance for over 10 years, but once I became pregnant, it only took a day of craving yogurt and I was hooked. I found that my lactose intolerance disappeared during my first pregnancy and has yet to return. The entire pregnancy, I craved milk shakes, ice cream, and yogurt. I assume this is largely brought on in part by the huge importance of calcium and vitamin D in human development.

Of course, I had some cravings and indulged in the occasional whole Italian-style pizza, greasy burgers, or salted caramel milkshake with no regrets. I encourage you to also give in a little and enjoy this time because meals will never be the same. The main objective here is balance. You will need to eat a proportional diet to ensure that that long list of nutrients is met and trust me when I say that your temptations will guide you. I typically skip the rice, bread, and most carbs, but while I was pregnant, I found myself needing that whole-grain toast or brown rice as fuel, but isn't that what carbs are for? That intuition will continue through breastfeeding I assure you!

Since I shared my unhealthy cravings, here are a few healthy options that gave me the energy I needed throughout pregnancy. Hunger pangs will strike and can cause lightheadedness. It will be important to keep some healthy "to-go" snacks to keep you and your baby fed, plus it helps to curb unhealthy cravings.

- Smoothies from Whole Foods (I found I couldn't grocery shop without it!)
- Whole grain peanut butter and jelly
- Greek yogurt with turmeric granola
- Grilled cheese
- Granola bars
- Fresh Fruit

In case you didn't get the memo, there are things you shouldn't eat due to the immature immune system of your sweet baby. And since your baby is not yet fully developed, they are often unable to fight off unusual bacteria that you can handle as a fully mature human. Here you can find a reminder of my least favorite things about pregnancy.

THE DO NOT EAT LIST:

- Raw eggs and seafood – No sushi or running eggs
- Undercooked meat – rare steaks

- Cold deli meats and cold bar salads - lunch meat or chicken salad
- Wine and alcohol – No explanation needed.
- Blue cheese and soft cheeses
- High mercury fish – Ahi Tuna, Shark, Swordfish
- Unpasteurized store-bought juices – Make them at home

Now that you've done all you can to nourish your little one, it's time to prepare for the grand appearance. Our ancestors were known to use the earth for healing and medicinal purposes. We as a people have become so disconnected from the earth, and yet it still provides us with our needs. For our body to initiate the labor process, we know for certain that our cervix must soften and thin out to open, also known as ripening. There are three naturally produced inducing remedies suggested by many midwives and doulas around the world. It has been documented that consuming these natural agents can aid in labor progression and promote a consistent labor experience. If you are being persuaded or coerced into induction, you can start inducing your labor with these earthly offerings before heading to your birthing space. Note that these must be used responsibly and preferably towards the end of pregnancy, as they can cause premature contractions.

EVENING PRIMROSE OIL

This oil comes from the evening primrose plant. It contains linolenic acid, gamma-linolenic acid, and vitamin E. It was initially used by Native Americans for medicinal purposes and can be taken orally or vaginally. According to the American Family Physicians, evening primrose oil may help the cervix soften and thin out in preparation for labor. Start by taking 500-2000 milligrams a day after 38 weeks.

RED RASPBERRY LEAF TEA

Red raspberry leaf tea is made from a plant native to Europe and parts of Asia. It is known for being the women's herb. Red raspberry leaves contain fragarine, a plant compound that helps tone and tighten muscles in the pelvic area. This tea is typically recommended for the second and third trimesters of pregnancy, and some women use the herbal remedy to help with nausea and vomiting in the first trimester as well. Red raspberry leaf tea has also been used to strengthen the uterus, improve labor outcomes, and prevent excessive bleeding after childbirth. It is even known to shorten labor. 1-3 cups a day should do it.

DATES

Dates are considered sacred fruit, especially in Islamic traditions. It is recommended during pregnancy and postpartum care in Islamic medical literature. In the Holy Koran, Allah instructs the Virgin Mary to consume date fruits when she gives birth to the prophet, Issa, peace will be upon him. The verse says, "And shake toward you, the trunk of the Palm tree, it will drop upon you, ripe fresh dates." Today, dates are still consumed traditionally during pregnancy and postpartum in regions of Asia and Africa. Not only is this sacred fruit packed with nutrients to provide energy, but it is also known to be an oxytocin receptor that produces more effective contractions[5]. It is encouraged that pregnant women consume 6 dates per day in the final 4 weeks of pregnancy to shorten and encourage cervical dilation. Tip: Dates can be a bit undesirable. Adding them to smoothies can help with consumption. Please note that these are not recommended for women who have been diagnosed with gestational diabetes due to their high sugar content.

Naturally wanting the best for my labor, I incorporated all three of the above starting at 36 weeks. I took the evening primrose orally, drank red raspberry leaf tea twice a day, and tried my best to consume as many dates as possible by incorporating them into my morning smoothie, adding to recipes, and occasionally just snacking on one. Due to the ability of these holistic supplements to induce labor, these serve best for low-risk pregnancies and when introduced in the third trimester.

ADJUSTMENTS AND ACUPRESSURE

Although acupressure is not rooted in Black culture, it has been practiced by many cultures, especially Chinese medicinal practices, for over 5,000 years. It is based on the concept of life energy which flows through "meridians" in the body. In treatment,

---

5   EBB birth, https://evidencebasedbirth.com/ebb-128-inducing-labor-with-castor-oil-and-dates/

physical pressure is applied to acupuncture points or ashi trigger points with the aim of clearing blockages in these meridians. Subsequently, it is known to relieve ailments within the body such as nausea, headaches, and low back pain. Acupressure is often coupled with chiropractic therapy.

My final physical preparation was through a few additional appointments with skilled therapeutic professionals. My doula recommended a chiropractor throughout the pregnancy but, being preoccupied with preparing my life in other ways, I put it off until the final 3 weeks when the demands of work slowed down and found additional free time.

The hormonal and physical changes you experience during pregnancy can affect your posture and alignment, which can lead to extreme discomfort in the final days of pregnancy. Adjustments designed to re-establish balance and alignment to your pelvis and spine will support your journey for a healthy and comfortable pregnancy, while also providing pain relief in your back, neck, hips, and joints. It can aid in positive outcomes for your birth experience by assisting expecting mothers with pelvis alignment. This creates adequate space in the birth canal for your baby to get in optimal birthing position, which reduces your risk of breech or posterior positioning subsequently reducing your risk of invasive birth and shorten labor time. My chiropractor experience was short but beneficial. I went in for my first evaluation and alignment at 37 weeks. After traveling by plane for months, I wasn't surprised to find that my pelvis and back were out of alignment. The Chiropractor recommended that I come in twice a week until I delivered and gave me a few aligning moves to practice at home. These appointments were partially covered by my insurance, so I decided to give it a shot. After a few visits, I noticed a real difference in prenatal yoga. I was able to do a few of the moves I struggled with before.

As far as the benefits I experienced the day of delivery with my newly aligned pelvis, I will never know for certain, but my active labor was short and I continued to have a comfortable pregnancy even at 39 weeks, and a properly positioned baby!

Mommy Tip: My Insurance provider had a "Healthy Baby" Program. I enrolled during my first trimester and each month, someone from the program contacted me to assess the progress of my pregnancy. In the end, I was rewarded with a $500 gift card for my participation. Be sure to research insurance programs to help offset additional preparation costs.

INDUCTION MASSAGES

An induction massage focuses on acupressure points found in the back to the legs, feet, and hands which can do several things. An induction massage can help release your sacrum and pelvic area to create more space for your baby to come down into your pelvis. Since physical touch is a key element, a massage can naturally raise your body's level of oxytocin and that hormone can bring on labor contractions. Many massage therapists swear by their ability to help jump-start labor when a mom-to-be is overdue, with their focus on certain pressure points to move labor along. Therapists will only perform this massage if you have reached 38 weeks.

I was 39 weeks and 4 days pregnant when I got my induction massage. At that point, I was doing any and everything I could to stay active, so I took the metro to my appointments. When I arrived, I met a sweet, older Latin woman who had performed many induction massages and was confident in her ability to recognize labor signs in a woman's body. About 30 minutes into my 60-minute massage, I started experiencing intense belly tightening and my body temperature started to rise. The therapist informed me that these were indeed labor contractions and assured me I would be in labor by the end of the weekend.

I continued to feel mild belly tightening and signs of early labor the remainder of the weekend. That Sunday evening, Mother's Day 2019, labor picked up. Sometime after dinner, I found myself in active labor which continued throughout the night. I welcomed a beautiful baby girl at 6:20 am the following morning.

To help you stay focused on your overall health throughout your pregnancy, I have included a checklist at the end of this chapter. See if you can do many of these if not all. It will help you to get one step closer to preparing your body and belly for your birth experience.

PREPARE THE BODY AND BELLY CHECKLIST:

- [ ] Participate regularly in Prenatal Yoga class
- [ ] Try a Barre class
- [ ] Check insurance for pregnancy programs
- [ ] Review pregnancy diet limitations

- [ ] Find the naturally prepared prenatal vitamins
- [ ] Create a plan to stay active
- [ ] Obtain items to naturally induce labor
- [ ] Keep healthy snacks readily available
- [ ] Track weight gain
- [ ] Sit on the birthing ball often
- [ ] Do birth ball exercises on YouTube
- [ ] Try Chiropractic Therapy
- [ ] Schedule an Induction Massage

Here, also, are some tips on how to prevent tearing during birth.

- [ ] Avoid an epidural
- [ ] Perineal massage
- [ ] Avoid episiotomy
- [ ] Warm Compress
- [ ] Coconut oil or another form of natural lubricant
- [ ] Breathe down while the baby is crowning. Try to sustain this throughout pushing
- [ ] Reduce your time pushing
- [ ] Push baby out while:
  - ◊ Kneeling
  - ◊ Hands & Knees
  - ◊ Side-Lying

7

CONNECT TO YOUR BABY AND YOUR SOUL

Throughout my pregnancy, I practiced mindfulness using a prenatal and postnatal birth meditation app on my phone. This app provided me with positive affirmations, breathwork, and soothing music that could transport me to another realm where I spoke with my unborn baby. To truly get in touch with your soul and your baby, you will need discipline, practice, and the ability to silence the outside world, and I can assure you that this will not come easily. It's like breathwork in yoga, you'll feel like you're not doing it correctly until the time comes when you have no other choice but to do it correctly, like when you're in a binded position and the only control you have left is the consistency of your breath and the power of your connection, and fear no longer becomes an option. This will be your final moment before meeting your baby. Believe me, you will find the strength to do whatever it takes to bring your beautiful baby earth-side.

For centuries, African culture has been deeply rooted in the power of spirituality and meditation. Many traditions and ancestral practices born out of enslavement often infuse Christianity with West African spiritual traditions to provide a more affirming and healing experience. Today, they are particularly attractive to Black women because traditional African spiritual beliefs honor and uplift the Black female body. Also, practicing customs from our ancestors drives us to connect with their strengths, and honor them as we navigate unsafe spaces such as our current medical landscape. We do this by creating rituals. Rituals serve as a gateway to the land of our ancestors and the spirit realm. It evokes sacredness and intentionality. Rituals anchor us to our community, give structure and meaning to life. By claiming strength, power, and rituals, we are more equipped to combat modern fears associated with pregnancy and settle in peace and trust.

As we discussed in previous chapters, fear is the enemy of unmedicated vaginal labor. This is because fear experienced during labor activates our primal fight-or-flight mechanism which then causes stress hormones called catecholamines to be released. The cascading effect is that this hormone causes the heart to quicken, forces blood to the arms and legs, and depletes blood flow to the uterus, creating uterine tension and hindering the labor process. It's been said that it is physically impossible for the body to be relaxed and in fight-or-flight mode simultaneously. This is also true for a woman who experiences fear during labor.

I stepped into my pregnancy with the strong belief that nature intended for women to give birth easily. By replacing fear with relaxation, a different set of chemicals come into play: oxytocin, prostaglandins (labor hormone), and endorphins combine to relax the muscles and create a sense of comfort. This trust in yourself and your body goes a long way; just think about mothers who plan to birth at home. According to the Midwives Alliance of North America, homebirths have a high rate of completed vaginal births (93%) and extremely positive breastfeeding rates of 97% up to 6 weeks postpartum. These women have chosen to put all their trust in their bodies and what their bodies are meant to do in the comfort of their home, removed from the fearmongering and pressure that leads to a cascade of interventions. The elimination of these pressures and distractions results in more peace and trust for the process.

Although I never took a full class on hypnobirthing, I would consider my birthing experience to be very much aligned with this practice. Hypnobirthing is a birthing method that uses self-hypnosis and relaxation techniques to help a woman feel prepared to give birth physically, mentally, and spiritually, and reduces her awareness of fear, anxiety, and pain during childbirth. This method is based on the work of Dr. Grantly Dick-Reed whom we discussed at the beginning of this book. His book, "Childbirth without Fear," identifies that no other animal species in the process of birth is associated with any suffering, pain, or agony.

As a result of staying in tune with my body and my baby, I did not consider pain medications, scream, or yell, check the clock, or doubt myself. I affirmed the ability of my body and baby to be able to work as one. I referred to my contractions as birth waves. I rested between birth waves. I visualized breathing my baby down the birth canal, and I envisioned my daughter being born. I was able to achieve this by practicing daily.

Meditation and spiritual connection did not only contribute to me remaining calm and peaceful throughout the labor process, but also to my daughter doing the same. She came out as the most peaceful and trusting baby girl. Today, I feel we have such a deep spiritual connection. During her infancy and early toddler years, I felt very in tune with her most basic needs, and even today, I feel confident knowing that I did everything in my power to bring her into this world, free of all medical interventions, into a peaceful setting with a mother who was present for every first moment. Although I understand that there are certainly many justifiable reasons for interventions, the key here is to condition your mind to trust your body to allow for a more instinctual birthing process. It may not be possible for every woman, but it is certainly possible for more women than those that are currently experiencing connected experiences. Disconnected birthing experiences are too widely known as the standard for Black women. If we do not empower our minds to trust and hear our bodies, we will be left with fewer people to listen to our needs and desires in the birthing room.

For mental preparation, I advise establishing a very intentional ritual around dispelling the thoughts of fear and pains surrounding birth. Take time out each day to meditate. This meditation should include holding affirmations that are aligned with you, your body, and your vision for your birth. They should be intentional and decode your present fears associated with birth. For instance, are you concerned about your baby's head crowning or the size of your baby? A good affirmation would be: My baby is the perfect size for my body.

Do these mediations in places around your home where you plan to labor. In your bed, on the couch, in the bathtub, or even in the baby nursery. If you are a visual person, write these affirmations around your home, or on your bathroom mirror, or the fridge. When the delivery day arrives, you will feel a sense of familiarity and calmness from your practice. You can find birth affirmations on whatever music streaming service you utilize. Take the time to listen to a few each day and find messages that are practical for you. As you listen, visualize your baby coming down the birth canal, out of your body, and into your arms. The more you practice, the more skilled you will become at eliminating fear, distractions and focusing on the labor. My partner joined in by often praying with me and creating his own mantras to help keep me on track. Whenever fear crept in, he would say, "She knows what to do," reminding me that babies are created with survival instincts too and that our strong baby girl planned to find her way into our arms just as much as we were hoping that she would.

This brings me to the topic of how to protect your soul. During your pregnancy, you will hear many birthing stories and start to notice patterns. People will try to project their fears and stories onto you. You will also notice, as your due date approaches, just how little is known about the unmedicated birthing process. Due to the overmedicalization of birth, you will get so many questions and comments pushing you in the exact direction you plan to avoid. Know that this is natural, and that people mean well, even if their advice is coming from a place of ignorance. It will be your duty to protect your energy and your future. You and your provider may have chosen to forgo cervix checks until necessary and this may be a foreign concept to a mother who was checked weekly leading up to her birth. Remember that your due date is just a calculation. Many babies come two weeks early or two weeks late, all of which can still occur without medication. People will give you unsolicited advice, don't take it personally or seriously. A male friend of ours suggested that I get induced before my actual due date. This is how common birth induction has become in our society.

The best thing you can do for yourself, and your family is to establish a plan to keep these influences away. This is the time to let the family know that you will reach out when something changes and then proceed to put your phone on "Do not disturb". This is also the time to distance yourself from mom friends with less-than-optimal birth experiences and reach out to your like-minded mom tribe; moms who are proud of their birthing experiences.

This is what I did, I surrounded myself with natural birthing mamas who reminded me that the birth I envisioned for me, and my baby, was obtainable. Women who championed for me and reminded me of what was possible. To be honest, I had to cut some mamas off temporarily because their experiences could potentially cloud my focus and make me doubt myself and my plans. There is power in consumption, in what you choose to consume or accept as a part of your story. When I heard stories from fellow mamas, I sympathized with these women, but deep down I knew that wasn't my story. I will share that I was classified as a low-risk pregnancy and healthy young, active woman, so my anticipated risks were minimal to start with. I also chose not to become impatient with the process and to trust that things would happen just as they should. There wasn't going to be any rush to check my dilation, no *"this baby needs to hurry up,"* or *"I'm over being pregnant."* Instead, I continued to enjoy every moment of preparing for the arrival of my baby girl.

At the end of this chapter, I have a beautiful letter written by my doula to my daughter. In the letter, she shares a vivid timeline of my daughter's personal birth story. I feel honored to pass down a positive birth story to my daughter, one that she will carry on her journey to motherhood. I hope that by sharing our birth experience, you will also have more insight into the possibilities of having a fully prepared birth and what it can look like for you. Below, I have included another checklist to help you get a few steps closer to connecting to your soul and your baby.

PREPARE THE BABY AND SOUL CHECKLIST:

- [ ] Practice your breathwork
- [ ] Give your contractions a positive name
- [ ] Choose affirmations for your labor and delivery
- [ ] Create a birth affirmation playlist
- [ ] Meditate daily
- [ ] Talk to your baby
- [ ] Visualize your birth experience
- [ ] Find a few like-minded women to check in with
- [ ] Read my Timeline of Childbirth

POSITIVE AFFIRMATIONS:

- I am enough for my baby.
- My baby is the perfect size for my body.
- I relax and my baby relaxes.
- My body is perfectly created for carrying and birthing my baby.
- I have the right to make decisions for my body and my baby.
- I will breathe my baby down and into my arms.
- I will surround myself with a positive tribe that advocates for the birth I see for me and my baby.
- I will not allow others to project their fears surrounding birth onto me and my journey.
- I inhale courage and exhale fear.
- My mind is at ease. I walk into birth with calm confidence, knowing that I can handle whatever comes my way.
- I choose to embrace the miracle of birth.
- I know I can deliver my baby naturally.
- I trust my instincts. I trust my body. I believe I can, and so I will.
- I trust the process of birth. My baby is healthy.
- My body is designed to do this. I trust the process and rhythm of birth.
- Each contraction brings me closer to my baby.
- I envision a peaceful birth. Pregnancy is not a medical condition. It is a beautiful yet customary part of life.

TIMELINE OF CHILDBIRTH JOURNEY BY FATIMA ABDULLAH

Nicole, Johnny, and Baby Alexandria Gwynn Bailey
Born Monday, May 13th, 2019 @ 6:20 am

Dear Ally,

My name is Fatima, and I was honored to be the doula on the journey that your parents took to help bring you earthside. I hope this timeline helps give you a glimpse into the day(s) leading up to your birth. I was lucky to have witnessed the love that your parents had for you and all the steps that they took to prepare for your arrival and make it the most peaceful and loving environment that it could be.

- Throughout their pregnancy, Nicole and Johnny did an amazing job preparing for your peaceful and gentle arrival into this world. They worked hard to find the right provider and doula, took childbirth and breastfeeding classes, and set themselves up in the best way possible.
- Once we met for our first prenatal in March 2019, I could tell how much love there was between your parents. They took this special time to discuss things together, to respect each other's opinions and preferences and I loved witnessing that amazing interchange. Topics like who would be present in the birth space, what kinds of words they preferred using to describe the birth process, how and when to move to the birth space. I was excited to be a witness to this love and intentionality that your parents put into

- bringing you, Ally, into this world, and into the deep love that they already had for you.
- Throughout the next few weeks of pregnancy, your momma, Nicole started incorporating daily pregnancy and birth affirmation and meditation sessions into her day, along with everything else she was doing. She was building her confidence in her birth and connecting with you daily through these moments.
- Around early May, Nicole started having early signs of her birthing time approaching. She and your dad were so excited and ready to meet you.
- On Mother's Day, Sunday, May 12th, 2019, I heard from Nicole around 5 pm, that she was having more birth signs. We knew this meant that things would happen soon, and we were excited. Nicole started feeling light birth waves but wasn't sure of them around 3 pm that day (which I found out about later) and she and Johnny decided to keep thinking positively and keep on going about with their day. That day they toured a possible new home open house and got back home where Momma Nicole cooked a delicious dinner. They ate around 6 pm that day and she noticed that she was still having her possible birth waves but thought it would still be a while.
- Around 11 pm, your loving daddy, Johnny, messaged me and wrote, "Hi! I'm fairly sure we're in the early phase of labor." I was excited to hear that and wanted to learn more. He let me know that things had started around 9 pm and he had set up a relaxing bath for Momma and was timing

the birth waves. "She's doing great so far." We talked about whether they felt like getting any sleep to see if they could save some energy for active labor and we waited.

- A little before 1 am, I reached out to see how things were going. Johnny let me know that Momma Nicole was 'handling it well... trying to sleep but they keep coming... birthing meditations playing to help." He mentioned that birth waves were about 8 minutes apart at this point. I was excited to hear that and knew that it meant this meant we were getting closer. I asked if they were ready for me to join them and around 1:30 am got the thumbs up to join.

- By 2:30 am I made it to your parents' place and found a beautifully peaceful sight. Nicole was in bed on her side, working through her powerful birth waves peacefully, with her Gentle Birth meditations playing quietly, dim lights in the hallway. Johnny was close by, giving her lots of gentle comfort touch and telling her how wonderful she was doing. Over the next hour, we kept the lights dim, and the birthing meditations and relaxing atmosphere going and tried a couple of different positions and worked on staying hydrated and comfortable. Nicole was working through her birth waves soooo amazingly, with strength and peace.

- Around 3:50 am, we moved out to the living room to work through some more birth waves, where it felt a little cooler and Nicole could try slightly different hand and knee/ curled positions. Just about an hour later, Nicole said, "She needs me to push." I was amazed that your momma was so in tune with you and her body, and I knew it was time to

119

go! We called Johnny from the bedroom and started getting things ready to go. Momma Nicole needed to use the bathroom one last time before we left, and there on the toilet, at around 5:20 am, her waters released with a splash into the toilet. We quickly headed out to the hospital and your daddy drove your momma quickly and calmly to the hospital, arriving by 5:45 am.

- Johnny left the car at the hospital door and Nicole and he walked into the hospital, like the strong parents they are.
- The hospital nurses checked your momma and found that she was 9 centimeters dilated with you so ready to be born! Momma was still maintaining her amazing strength and peaceful demeanor. She got onto a hands and knees position on the hospital bed and gently breathed you out with a few gentle breaths.
- At 6:20 am, you were born into this world, with your loving daddy looking on, soooo excited to meet your little face. Momma breathed one last calm breath and released you into this world, right into your Midwife Ilana and Daddy Johnny's waiting arms.
- Your momma was so happy to finally meet you, and as you went into her arms and she saw your eyes, she said, "I've been waiting for these eyes. I've been waiting to meet these eyes." It was the most beautiful and loving meeting I have seen and the most beautiful and peaceful birth.

PART 3:
WELCOME TO MOTHERHOOD

The moment you've been waiting for has finally arrived! It's the day to hold life's precious gift in your arms, to care for every morning, noon, and night. Although the magic of childbirth has been experienced, we still have a whirlwind of recovery and adjustments necessary to get you back to optimal productivity and, most importantly, to enjoy the joys of motherhood. I pray that with my guidance and your strength, you were able to get your baby earth-side just as you envisioned. If not, it's ok, I'm sure you put forth your best effort and your intentions are in

> Birth is not only about making babies. Birth is about making mothers—strong, competent, capable mothers who trust themselves and know their inner strength.
> —Barbara Katz Rothman

the right place. And more importantly, you had the confidence to advocate not only for your baby but for YOU! In this chapter, we will explore what happens once your baby makes its grand entrance into this world. We will talk about breastfeeding and its many challenges and how to overcome them; postpartum preparation and care, and how to establish and adjust to your new normal.

8

POSTPARTUM PREPARATION AND CARE

Women can easily neglect their physical, mental, emotional, and spiritual well-being during this time when living in the West. This is mostly because the demands of life, according to Western culture, do not stop long enough for new mothers to properly take care of themselves.

Giving birth was originally designed to be a cultural, biological, and social experience for the mother, it was a rite of passage for any woman choosing to partake in the miracle of life. As such, certain cultural rituals and traditions preserved amongst women communities have provided support to the recovery of new mothers for centuries. In African and Caribbean traditions, both stand firm on making sure that women rest after giving birth while others tend to their homes. In some African nations, there are confinement traditions, which vary from country to country. During these confinement periods, mother and baby are quarantined for anywhere from 10 to 40 days while friends and relatives provide the family with meals and care for other children. Many women in Latin American countries like the Dominican Republic and Mexico observe "la cuarentena," which translates to "quarantine." La cuarentena, it is believed, is the 40 days it takes for the uterus to return to its normal size and form after giving birth. During La Cuarentena, relatives pitch in to cook, clean, and take care of the kids. Many Latinas believe that strictly following cuarentena guarantees good health in old age and guards against maladies like headaches.

The common thread across these cultures is that postpartum care is considered a delicate time that restores strength to the mother and protects the newborn against illness by caring for the mother and loving the newborn. They understand that although the baby is now outside of its mother's body, they were still connected. This disruption of the physical connection requires time to adjust, and some sensitivity awareness, as mother and baby are still very much bonded by necessity. They also understand that after birth, a mother will experience the time of "Mamatoto", a word in Swahili, which means "mother-baby". This is described as the interdependent physical, spiritual, and energy bond still flowing through mother and baby as one. The mother-baby physiology is designed for an unmedicated vaginal birth. When our birth experiences take other directions, there are unfinished processes that require another level of healing. This is why the recovery period looks different for every woman, depending on various factors, and is primarily based on what happened during birth.

The fact that women require postpartum healing is nothing new. We have all known and observed this for centuries. The problem is that this knowledge has not been integrated into our current cultural and social settings.

The good news is that the importance of postpartum care is returning to many conversations amongst birth workers. You will find postpartum doulas providing support and restorative rituals for mothers. This is because the time following the birth of your baby should be used to restore your strength through rest, nutrients, and rituals to help you find healing, and to bond with your newborn. This is a time to accept family support and allow lengthy visits to make space for restoration. You may be surprised at who supports you and how relieved you will be when you get that much-needed support. If your extended family support is limited, you can take advantage of a postpartum doula. Postpartum doulas provide not only the emotional support often needed after such a big passage, but breastfeeding guidance, newborn care, self-care tips, meals, family transitions, and so much more. They may even provide placenta encapsulation.

This period is now being more commonly referred to as the fourth trimester. The fourth trimester goes unrecognized as an important part of women's health care, according to Kimberly Ann Johnson, the author of The Fourth Trimester. As a new mother, I now have a newfound respect for the power of sharing information, shedding light on complex or uncomfortable parts of the motherhood journey. I will take you through a few of my most intimate moments during my fourth trimester, I hope they give you strength and guidance, and awareness that allows you to transition with more grace and ease.

One thing that I vividly recall, following labor, was not being able to control my bladder for the first few hours. It amazed me to find out that I was numb down below without having had an epidural or any type of medication. I discovered that when a mother is left to labor undisturbed, she might experience what is called the Fetal Ejection Reflex. This is when the body expels your baby with no real effort from the birthing mother. Her body simply does it on its own, naturally. It's like a sneeze!

After giving birth, the nurse gave me ibuprofen and a stool softener which helped when the numbness wore off and assisted with my first bowel movement. I dreaded the thought of tearing and was on edge as I waited to be assessed. My midwife did a quick examination and found that I had no tears. This may be the result of several things; I believe one of those things for me was choosing to give birth on all fours with my arms hanging over the hospital headboard. This wasn't something I asked permission to do or even planned for, my body simply moved into the position that seemed most comfortable and, thank goodness for this instinct because although I felt a wave of exhaustion from laboring all night, I found the courage to listen to my body and my baby one more time. I recall asking if it was time to push and the midwife said yes but to wait for my next contraction to push. Sure enough, my next contraction came, and I took three or four deep breaths and exhaled down my body. I recall my hubby encouraging the midwife to continue pouring coconut oil over my vaginal opening and within a few more minutes my baby was being handed to me through my legs. We immediately did skin-to-skin contact and our first latch, which takes time to perfect. At the end of this section, I have included the steps I took to prevent tearing during childbirth. This is particularly important because of all the women I talked to, no one told me there was a possibility of not tearing. That there were ways to ease into the crowning process. To be quite honest, the biggest threat to pushing is the lack of sensation and distractions.

Keep in mind that during the first few weeks, it will be pertinent that you take it slowly and take good care of yourself. You have been through substantial changes, physically, mentally, and hormonally. The old wife's tale advises five days in bed, five days on the bed, and five days around the bed. Ideally, that means 15 days of not leaving your room, keeping your legs closed, and minimizing your moments. This will allow crucial healing of your pelvis floor and restoration of your pelvis fibers. Your internal organs will also need to settle back in place and recalibrate. After giving birth vaginally, you will bleed for about 2-3 weeks, experience soreness in your belly, feel contractions as your uterus works to retract back to its normal size, and experience vaginal sensitivity or soreness.

As postpartum care becomes more commonly discussed, a much-needed market to meet women's health needs has emerged. You will find many new items on the market to support some of your postpartum ailments. I will never forget when a fellow mommy told me to make sure I get a diaper for myself, I was in total disbelief, but at least I was now aware. Surprisingly, this information was not shared with me by my midwives, doula, or even my mother, instead, it was shared with me by a new mom friend I'd made on social media. That feminine adult diaper came in handy those first few days following birth, as well as the Peri refillable bottle, perineal spray, and an overnight pad. I used the peri bottle when I had to urinate until I noticed the swelling and sensitivity had reduced. I was afraid to use the bathroom without the relief that the peri bottle provided. I also replaced the hospital padsicle with the perineal spray once I felt the swelling had subsided. I used my feminine adult diaper merely because the hospital ones weren't the most secure fit, but they will do the job. This regimen will last for at least 2-3 weeks, depending on the type of birth and recovery your body requires.

Other than that, your days should only be filled with resting, healing, and bonding. Your daily routine should include snuggling up with your newborn, nursing often (this helps your uterus shrink back), keeping your body nourished, and simply caring for your new baby and yourself. Instead of engaging in chores, start self-care rituals, such as a sitz bath and letting go of heavy demands to refill yourself. There will be plenty of late nights and early mornings for the next 12-24 months, and never-ending chores to last you a lifetime. This is the time to avoid housework and get familiar with your infant workload and the new you! When friends and family ask how they can support you, let them know to drop off meals, assist with chores, pick things up from the store, and anything that will lighten the load for you and your family during this adjustment period. Try to embody the tradition of 40 days if possible. This will give your body some time to heal and gain an understanding of how to begin to process your new identity as a mother. I know this can be challenging, but even as you reenter life, try to start simple. Motherhood is like no other life experience you've ever had.

I was lucky to have my mother and sister come and support us for the first few weeks of postpartum. They provided meals and completed household duties like laundry and cleaning. Friends brought over homecooked meals, takeout, or even sent items through delivery services. You will need all the help you can get even if that doesn't include infant care. You may be cautious about others caring for your newborn, but you can certainly find other ways for them to provide support to keep your home running somewhat efficiently.

My doula specialized in postpartum healing for mothers, so she was able to bundle that into my postpartum care package which included homemade lactation cookies, energy snack balls, nourishing postpartum soups and teas, and healing sitz baths. These items enhanced my healing experience since they were readily available to keep me going or relaxed when needed. This is extremely important, especially since much of the attention is going to revolve around your newborn. As new mothers, we tend to neglect the attention our bodies deserve as we make room in our lives for our babies – by creating nurseries, new routines, develop new work lives, etc. I encourage you to identify these feelings early and often, do not let them go ignored.

Our healing is multifaceted, our nutritional intake is just as important in the fourth trimester as it was in the first. Our bodies crave whole foods all the time, but these cravings increase when our strength is depleted and we're actively losing blood. It also increases when we find ourselves healing from any tears or surgeries. For example, your body will be in wound repair mode following childbirth, your muscles will crave the protein needed to repair stressed tissues. One of the best sources of protein for childbirth recovery is salmon since it is full of omega-3 fatty oils, which have been proven to reduce inflammation. It has even been linked to managing stress and preventing postpartum depression.

Here is a list of nutritional sources for postpartum healing. These will provide your body with the antioxidants, bodybuilding, and mineral-rich nutrients it needs to aid in recovery and to give you that boost of energy you will need to meet the new demands of motherhood. Although fast food is always tempting, I encourage you to make balanced choices to support your necessary recovery. While you are going through this list, keep in mind that diet is also linked to the quality and quantity of your milk production[6].

- Avocados: Are an excellent source of polyunsaturated and monounsaturated fat, which helps the body absorb fat-soluble vitamins that feed the brain and assist the nervous system.
- Bananas: Rich in potassium, vitamin B6, vitamin C, manganese, fiber, and protein, this fruit also moderates blood sugar levels and aids the digestive system.
- Beets: With essential nutrients such as B vitamins, magnesium, boron, and iron, beets are blood builders, and they balance cholesterol levels and help maintain a healthy cardiovascular system.
- Blueberries (and other berries): Berries are loaded with fiber, manganese, vitamin K, and vitamin C. They are an

---

[6] Information obtained from Fourth Trimester book, By Kimberly Ann Johnson.

extremely high antioxidant food, helping the body neutralize free radicals and repair DNA damage.
- Cherry tomatoes: A great source for vitamin C, vitamin A, and B6. They may help repair cellular damage and protect against osteoporosis and skin damage.
- Dandelion greens: Rich in Vitamin B complex as well as minerals such as choline, magnesium, boron, and iron. These can also aid the digestive system, liver, and gallbladder.
- Figs: This stone fruit will help lower high blood pressure and they are loaded with potassium, essential minerals, and a high density of phenolic antioxidants. They protect the heart and regulate kidney and liver functions.
- Mango: The most effective antioxidant, mangoes are loaded with vitamin C, pectin, and fiber. They help to lower serum cholesterol levels and boost the immune system and are alkalizing to the whole body due to the content of tartaric acid, malic acid, and citric acid.
- Papaya: Containing papain, an enzyme that helps digest proteins, papayas are loaded with antioxidants such as vitamin C, flavonoids, vitamin B, folate, and pantothenic acid, which help reduce inflammation.
- Pears: These are mineral-rich in magnesium, folate, calcium, and iron, as well as high in vitamin C and fiber, which aids the digestive system.
- Persimmon: An excellent antioxidant and a source for beta-carotene and vitamin C, this fruit also contains compounds that are anti-inflammatory and anti-hemorrhagic.

They are rich in minerals, including copper, which helps build red blood cells.

- Pomegranate: A great source for vitamin B complex, minerals, vitamin C, and antioxidants, pomegranates also improve circulation and help build immunity.

NUTS, SEEDS, AND GRAINS (PLANT-BASED PROTEINS)

- Almonds: Are protein-rich and contain calcium and manganese and are also anti-inflammatory.
- Cashews: These nuts are rich in vitamin E and K, selenium, antioxidants, and minerals.
- Walnuts: These nuts contain essential fatty acids, protein, and minerals.
- Cacao nibs: An excellent source of magnesium, an essential mineral for the respiratory and circulatory system, as well as a source of essential minerals and phytonutrients.
- Chia seeds: These are the most bio-available protein source, helping the body stay hydrated and moisturized from within.
- Hemp seeds: These seeds contain omega fatty acids, protein, and fiber, as well as having anti-inflammatory and antioxidant properties.
- Millet: This seed is rich in protein, fiber, and minerals, helping to regulate blood sugars.
- Pumpkin seeds: These are mineral-rich, as well as having antioxidant and anti-inflammatory properties.

- Sunflower seeds: Full of protein, this good carbohydrate is also a mineral-rich choice.
- Quinoa: This grain is protein-rich, full of fiber, and has anti-inflammatory and antioxidant properties.
- Wild rice blend or brown rice: These types of rice are full of protein, fiber, and good carbohydrates.

PROTEINS

- Fish
- Seafood
- Grass-fed animal products are the ideal choice.
- Chicken
- Eggs
- Bone broth
- Chicken breasts or thighs
- Turkey sausage
- Duck
- Bacon
- Salmon
- Raw cheese
- Full fat yogurt
- Chickpeas
- Black beans

BEVERAGES AND LIQUIDS

- Almond milk
- Oat milk
- Hemp milk
- Fennel tea
- Chamomile tea
- Raspberry leaf tea
- Roasted dandelion tea

HEALTHY FATS

Fats are vital for proper brain function and absorbing nutrients, which is why we feel good when eating healthy fats. All good for you, the difference is in fat composition.

- Duck Fat
- Olive oil
- Butter
- Avocado
- Coconut oil
- Ghee Butter

SWEETENERS

Postpartum, low glycemic index, and stable blood sugar levels will help your hormones recalibrate. Here are some options for natural sweeteners.

- Local raw honey: Honey contains essential nutrients and is medicine. Local honey is a natural antibiotic and is anti-fungal and anti-viral.
- Maple syrup: Mineral-rich and low glycemic, this is a perfect choice for a sweetener.
- Agave

As with prior chapters, I'm providing you with a few resources to assist with your postpartum transition. Although nothing quite prepares you for what's on the other side of pregnancy, I will try my best to ease your transition with a list of things that kept me grounded and supported during my postpartum period.

- **Postpartum Plan**
  ◊ Having a postpartum plan will help you address your most important needs during a time of great transition. This will also allow you and your family to rest while having access to nourishing food, physical touch, family support, and fresh air. Here are a few things you and your family can discuss to be more prepared for the newborn weeks.
  ◊ Notify Family and Friends
    - Create a list and action plan for notifying family and friends about your new arrival.
  ◊ Visitors
    - Who do you want to visit for the first 3 days?
    - Who do you want to visit for the first 2 weeks?
    - Who do you want to visit for the first month?
  ◊ Rest
    - How will you manage nightly feedings?
    - How will you manage nightly diaper changes?
    - Where will you put the bassinet?
    - Who do you trust to watch your baby while you nap?
    - How will you create space to nap during the day when you have visitors?
    - How will you create space to step away from technology and devices, such as laptops and cell phones to be present?
  ◊ Food

- List 3 of your favorites and/or your partner's favorite meals. You can share this with family who offers to cook for you.
- List 3 balanced snacks you enjoy.
- Organize a meal train or delegate someone to handle this for you.
- Make a list of your favorite local restaurants and your typical order.

◊ Companionship
- Who can you call for newborn or breastfeeding advice?
- Who can you call to keep you company while on maternity leave?
- Whose mothering views align with yours?
- Who is knowledgeable with local health resources or women centers?
- Go for a walk as a new family.
- Schedule a first family outing with your newborn and partner.

◊ Wellness Support
- Make a list of resources.
- Lactation support
- Pelvis Remediation Specialist
- Postnatal Yoga
- Chiropractor
- Massage therapist
- Housekeeper
- Postpartum Doula

- Night Nurse
- Local Breastfeeding Support Groups
◊ New mom support groups
  - Mommy and Me exercise groups
◊ Filling Your Soul
  - Make a list of books you want to read.
  - Subscribe to a podcast you want to get caught up on
  - Find uplifting shows or movies to watch.
  - Keep a journal.
  - Start a new project.
◊ Partner
  - Revisit your love languages.
  - Schedule the first date after your baby
  - Secure a babysitter.
  - Talk about the birthing experience.
  - Discuss current fears about parenthood.
  - Be open and honest about your new needs.

I have also gathered a list of items for your postpartum kit that will aid with some of the physical healing processes.

- Peri bottle
- Herbal perineal spray
- Feminine diapers
- Overnight pads
- Shapewear
- Stool softener
- Ibuprofen
- Herbal Sitz bath (homemade or store-bought)

WARNING SIGNS

While this is a beautiful, transformative moment for you, I want to also equip you with a list of things to watch out for to spot after-birth complications.

- Heavy Bleeding
- Fever
- Weakness
- Vision problems
- Severe headaches
- Severe pain in abdominals
- Swelling of legs
- Fast breathing
- Bad odor

If you experience any of these things, seek medical attention immediately. These may be a sign of blood clots, infections, or eclampsia. This is where choosing providers that respect you and listen to you comes into play. I hope by using the care provider interview questions in Chapter 4, that you have established a strong relationship with the right provider for you.

9

BREASTFEEDING WHILE BLACK

The origin of Black women breastfeeding in this country is not an appealing one. Since slavery, there have been legal, political, and societal factors that have routinely denied Black women the means to choose how to feed their babies.

> The exploitation and devaluing of Black families set the tone for a significant breastfeeding gap in America.

As if ripping Black mothers from their young and forcing them to work long hours on plantations while selling their children and killing or torturing their husbands wasn't enough, some plantation owners banned Black mothers from breastfeeding because they believed it was a contraceptive and they didn't want any delay in the breeding of more slave labor. Other plantation owners forced Black mothers to breastfeed their white children instead. These women became known as "wet nurses". The exploitation and devaluing of Black families set the tone for a significant breastfeeding gap in America.

Meanwhile, Africans believe that breastfeeding facilitates a strong bond between a mother and her child. Traditionally, it is the primary method of infant feeding in African culture, and many pregnant mothers looked forward to breastfeeding their newborns. Some Africans have a strong belief in the power of breastmilk; they believe that a woman is capable of blessing or casting a spell on a child with its power. Babies were often breastfed from the time they were born until they turned 2 years old or beyond. In ancient Egyptian times, breastfeeding was a religious obligation. New mothers were to breastfeed for the first six months and, if the mother died or was not capable for any reason, a wet nurse was secured. In both cases, breastfeeding is the ideal nutritional choice for the infant.

Unfortunately, the combination of slavery, racism, intergenerational trauma, and white privilege, as was previously discussed in Section 1 of this book, has made breastfeeding a luxury in the United States, thus denying Black mothers this powerful introduction into motherhood. According to national data, 83 percent of White mothers and 82 percent of Latinx mothers report ever attempting to breastfeed, while 66 percent of Black mothers report ever trying. Only 37 percent of low-income Black women even initiate breastfeeding. This gap continues to extend with systematic oppression and a lack of implemented maternity leave standards.

This is because social constructs make working and nursing fundamentally inharmonious. With 80% of Black mothers as breadwinners compared to 50% of White mothers, we often find ourselves back at work earlier than our White counterparts, making breastfeeding a tough feat without ample support and resources. White privilege has detached the long history of Black slaves and wet nurse expertise in breastfeeding and accredited white women for America's breastfeeding culture. It currently stands that flexibility, financial security, structural support, and resources are key components for breastfeeding in America. Making it more of a privilege instead of women's rights. By 6 months, only 35% of Black women still breastfeed compared to 56% White mothers and 51% Latinx mothers. Black infant formula use is significantly higher than White and Latinx infants and this is hardly a coincidence. Formula companies and the USDA have conspired to target Black mothers as their main consumers by offering free samples and preying on poor mothers through WIC programs, hospital partnerships, and pediatrician's offices. Instead of encouraging and providing resources for breastfeeding and postpartum anxiety, they are creating and maintaining a loyal consumer base, through the calculated exploitation of Black mothers. The USDA's priority is to aid in fueling the economy and to ensure that excess resources are utilized, not to reduce diabetes rates, reduce sudden infant death incidents or promote healthy weight for Black mothers or babies. The precise mission of the USDA states: *"We provide leadership on food, agriculture, natural resources, rural development, nutrition, and related issues based on public policy, the best available science, and effective management. We have the vision to provide economic opportunity through innovation, helping rural America to thrive; to promote agriculture production that better nourishes Americans while also helping feed others throughout the world; and to preserve our Nation's natural resources through conservation, restored forests, improved watersheds, and healthy private working lands."*

So, it should not come as a surprise that excess corn, milk, and soy are being dumped into baby formulas and that the USDA is the largest consumer of baby formula. Most formulas are highly produced products that are essentially babies' gateways to poor eating habits and processed foods. The USDA purchases a large supply through rebates to be given out to new mothers, who are sleep deprived, healing, and adjusting to a new normal. The WIC program does not distribute formula or breastfeeding education based on individual circumstances, but rather for six months, regardless of need. No questions are asked, and no additional support is given. This aids in the disproportionately low rates of breastfeeding mothers in the WIC program. Only 14.5% of mothers receiving WIC report breastfeeding exclusively for up to 6 months. The USDA can support formula companies and the agriculture industry by creating captive consumers by exploiting the vulnerable new Black mother.

You may be wondering why I just gave you an economics and history lesson. It's because breastfeeding is not just a preference, it is a form of activism. Here you are, with the power to break a generational curse, to deny a form of capitalism from entering your nursery, and to counter the exploitation of our communities. I know entering motherhood is overwhelming and there will be moments to consider what works for you, your family, and your baby, but I must remind you of the power of choice and knowledge. The system is not set up to create more healthy Black lives, it's set up to create more dependency and generate more revenue.

"Breastfeeding is the closest thing the world has to a magic bullet for child survival," states UNICEF. On a global scale, several studies link low breastfeeding rates to high infant mortality.

> Breastfeeding is not just a preference; it is a form of activism.

Of the twenty-six wealthiest and most industrialized nations, the United States has the highest rate of infant mortality. The numbers again show that the rate is twice as high for Black infants compared to white infants. The combination of racial disparities and related health issues looming in the Black communities make this a form of oppression.

Food oppression is a cooperative effort between the government and the food agriculture or pharmaceutical industries that lead to health disparities intersecting race, class, and gender. We do have the power to undo some of this oppression by choosing to breastfeed our young in hopes of establishing a healthier future. With the Black community constantly being plagued by higher rates of health disparities, we must start taking preventative methods into our own hands. One huge step we can take is to breastfeed our children first, this allows them to build a stronger foundation for better outcomes.

Breast milk contains antibodies that are passed along to your baby which helps them to fight off infection and disease. Breastfeeding reduces the risk of suffering from over sixty-five different conditions, including ear, respiratory, blood infections, SIDS, cancer, asthma, diarrhea, diabetes, impaired speech, language, and brain development. From a strictly health-focused approach, baby formula is no match for breastmilk. And although formula may serve as a replacement when needed to combat various personal challenges, it will never serve as an equal replacement. I felt like a superwoman knowing that my body was able to produce such a powerful guard for my new baby to navigate the world with me. From experience, I can firmly state that I breastfed for 14 months, and my baby girl was only sick one time.

Having a sick baby is no fun, in fact here are a few statistics that will keep you going on those long days and nights of breastfeeding:

- **Respiratory tract infections:** Exclusive breastfeeding for more than 4 months reduces the risk of hospitalization for these infections by up to 72%.
- **Colds and infections:** Babies exclusively breastfed for 6 months may have up to a 63% lower risk of getting serious colds and ear or throat infections.
- **Gut infections:** Breastfeeding is linked with a 64% reduction in gut infections, seen for up to 2 months after breastfeeding stops.
- **Intestinal tissue damage:** Feeding preterm babies breast milk is linked with around a 60% reduction in the incidence of necrotizing enterocolitis.
- **Sudden infant death syndrome (SIDS):** Breastfeeding is linked to a 50% reduced risk after 1 month, and a 36% reduced risk in the first year.

- **Allergic diseases:** Exclusive breastfeeding for at least 3–4 months is linked with a 27–42% reduced risk of asthma, atopic dermatitis, and eczema.
- **Celiac disease:** Babies who are breastfed at the time of first gluten exposure have a 52% lower risk of developing celiac disease.
- **Inflammatory bowel disease:** Babies who are breastfed may be roughly 30% less likely to develop childhood inflammatory bowel disease.
- **Diabetes:** Breastfeeding for at least 3 months is linked to a reduced risk of type 1 diabetes (up to 30%) and type 2 diabetes (up to 40%).
- **Childhood leukemia:** Breastfeeding for 6 months or longer is linked with a 15–20% reduction in the risk of childhood leukemia.

As parents, we want the best for our children; whether that's financial security, educational preferences, or equal opportunities, but let's ensure that good health is included in all the things we want for our children. Health disparities can be reduced by setting a new standard for our children's relationship with food. In efforts to diminish disproportionate health issues in our communities, we should reduce the amount of high sugar and processed formulas, setting a poor palate foundation for our Black infants.

Some benefits and preventive measures derived from breastfeeding for babies include the following:

- Promotes healthy weight gain and reduces the risk of childhood obesity.
- Produces leptin and healthy gut bacteria vital for managing appetite and fat storage.
- Breastfed babies learn to self-regulate their food intake much sooner than formula-fed babies. This sets the tone for healthy eating habits.
- Breastfed babies often have higher emotional intelligence, IQ scores, and fewer behavioral or learning problems.

For mothers, the benefits include:

- Mothers who breastfeed have lower risks of postpartum depression.
- Breastfeeding for more than one year is linked to a 28% lower risk of breast and ovarian cancer. It has also been linked to a reduced risk of several other diseases.
- Saves time and money! You don't have to worry about buying or mixing formula, warming up bottles, or calculating your baby's daily needs.
- Some mothers see a huge delay in their menstruation. I did not experience this at all. I credit this to my baby loving her sleep.

Like so many women, I heard the gamut of issues associated with the duration and initiation of breastfeeding. They ranged from, 'it hurts,' 'your milk dries up,' 'it's best to pump as soon as possible,' to, 'it's a burden to be the only partner doing night feedings,' and, 'not all babies latch.' Again,

I had to remove fear, move with affirmations, and channel my ancestors. I reminded myself that all civilizations originally relied on breast milk to thrive, so again as was stated for birth, this was not meant to be a painful process and it is entirely instinctive.

I nursed my daughter within minutes of her being born and, of course, neither one of us knew what we were doing yet. That's right, breastfeeding takes practice. It will take time for mommy and baby to figure it out, but with the right information and support, almost everyone can breastfeed. I laugh each time I see a picture of that first 24 hours trying to breastfeed because I look utterly dumbfounded. The midwife passed her to me with the umbilical cord still intact to rest on my chest and instinctively she turned for nourishment. Babies will naturally seek out your nipple. The next step is teaching them how to position their chin and nose for a successful latch. This will take time, so please don't be hard on yourself. I made sure to meet with the hospital lactation consultant a few times during her rounds. It helped me to gain some confidence while learning a few tricks to get my daughter to latch properly. During this time, we hadn't quite mastered the traditional cradle nursing position, so the lactation consultant suggested the football hold. It ended up helping us latch until we were comfortable doing other positions.

Once the latch is perfected, breastfeeding is one of the most harmonious and rewarding moments of motherhood. That feeling of knowing you can effortlessly solve all your baby's dilemmas with an intimate connection of feeding and cuddling is priceless. The look of content and satisfaction on your newborn's face will warm your heart and you will cherish these moments, the simple days when all your baby ever wanted was mommy's milk.

BREASTFEEDING CHALLENGES

So, let's unpack this pain associated with breastfeeding. The day you give birth, your milk has not come in yet, instead, you will be producing colostrum, which will meet your baby's needs until the milk comes in. This can take about 3-4 days. During this time, you may need to ice your breast and take warm showers with a warm washcloth on your chest, this will soothe the discomfort. This is honestly a very temporary discomfort, and I would describe it more as tenderness than actual pain. No reason to jump ship. If the pain continues, try adjusting your baby's latch, it's likely their little mouth is having a hard time taking enough into their mouth for a comfortable and efficient latch. It's important to seek help quickly to ensure you're able to establish a good milk supply.

When your milk finally comes in, you will know! You may leak or the milk drunk look on your infant's face will tell you. Your breast will begin to feel relieved each time you nurse. Babies do solely survive on milk at this point and rely on your ability to know when they need feedings. I used a Baby feeding mobile app for the first few weeks to track feedings and diaper changes. This will help you establish what is normal. The first few days are extremely intense. Newborns need to be fed every 2-3 hours or 8-10 times a day, add in the diaper changes and you have little time for anything else. While I did nurse often, I did not wake my baby up for nursing. I followed the motto that says not to wake a sleeping baby. Please use your best judgment and pediatrician's guidance to make an informed decision regarding waking your newborn for feedings.

Once we had the rhythm of nursing, there were only a few other times when I felt anything I would classify as pain. I did get a few clogged ducts during my time nursing. Common culprits of clogged ducts: birth control, Benadryl (I was stung by a bee and ended up swollen like a watermelon.), baby sleeping through the night, insufficient pumping, dehydration and not wearing the right bra. It typically started with warning signs, the baby complaining of not getting enough milk (crying), and my nipple beginning to throb from excessive sucking. Next thing I knew I would have some type of discoloration and lump on my breast wherever the clogged duct was located. The best thing to do is unclog this duct immediately. It can be extremely uncomfortable if you're outside the home. Get home as soon as you can and follow the instructions below:

REMOVING A CLOGGED DUCT:

1. Apply heat: warm showers, heating pads (home crafted or store-bought)
2. Use gravity: Nurse in different positions that allow your breast to hang down to encourage the clog to flow.
3. Massage: Try to loosen up clogs with a hand massage.

4. Nipple balm: This is a great time to use nipple balm. The ingredients will soothe irritated nipples and help avoid friction from pumping.
5. Pump often: After nursing, try pumping to see if you can get any additional milk out. I would often leave the pump on the pre-let down setting when I was clogged to allow for more stimulation.
6. Take a break: You may feel like nothing is helping because your breast is sore. But your breast can still be sore even if the duct is unclogged. So, don't overdo it. Try the steps above for no longer an hour with nursing and/or pumping then give yourself a break.
7. Apply cold: Place an ice pack on sore nipples during your break.
8. Repeat: I would repeat this no more than 2-3 times a day.
9. Supplements: If you find yourself having frequent clogged ducts due to being on birth control or the occasional bottle of wine like myself. I highly suggest getting a supplement, like milk thistle that helps with milk flow and production.
10. Drink more water.

Besides the occasional hiccup, breastfeeding is not painful. It is certainly not consistently painful. Pain is often associated with an issue: such as a clogged duct, infection, or improper latching, in other words, there are solutions, and you can get back to pain-free nursing in no time.

I know the first weeks can be difficult. One thing I did was to ensure that my birth team was a good resource for breastfeeding questions. My doula, although she was not a licensed lactation consultant, at the time, she had nursed 4 children of her own. She checked in periodically and answered any questions or concerns I had surrounding breastfeeding. We also identified a pediatrician who was a licensed lactation consultant.

If you are experiencing additional struggles with breastfeeding, please reach out to a local lactation consultant or a postpartum doula before giving up. Remember that you do not have to figure this all out on your own. Whether bottle-feeding or getting your baby to latch, here are a few tips to guide you as you get started on your breastfeeding journey.

IS BABY GETTING ENOUGH MILK?

As a new mother, one of the most important things you can learn is whether your precious baby is getting enough milk. There are more than two ways to figure this out:

1. By noticing the deep rhythmic drop of your baby's jaw as they suck and swallow your milk.
2. The frequency with which your baby passes urine and stools.
3. A baby who is getting enough milk will be awake and active during feeding time. If your baby is quickly losing interest in breastfeeding, take a closer look at their latch or investigate holistic ways to increase your production.
4. Your baby should be waking up for about 8-10 feedings by the end of the first week.

This is a common concern for most mothers, often leading them to pump too soon or introduce formula. Remember newborn's tummies are very small and it doesn't take much for you to make few minor adjustments to ensure you're producing enough milk for your baby to thrive. At the end of this chapter, you find 8 holistic ways to increase your milk supply.

PUMPING

There are several breast pumps on the market created to fit your lifestyle and schedule. They range from free (covered by insurance thanks to the affordable care act) to $500. There is one for every budget. They can be manual, rechargeable, battery-operated, cord-free, and even wearable.

Here's a list of options:

Manual Pumps – This is for the occasional pumper or compact pump for a night out when you don't have access to an outlet. This pump is hand-powered and usually requires you to pump a lever or hand express. I have used this as a backup in an emergency to provide relief.

Electric Pumps – This is for the regular pumpers and the working mamas. This gives you a choice of suction modes and pumping styles. Your insurance will cover the hospital-grade pumper and typically offers the option to pay additional for a cordless one. This was my go-to pumping option. I had a rechargeable hospital-grade breast pump that I used day and night. I highly suggest replacing parts to keep the integrity of the milk and the efficiency of the pump. Duckbill valves should be replaced every 4-12 weeks, while flanges and milk collection bottles should be replaced every 6 months.

Wearable pumps – This is the priciest option although it is also great for the mom who plans to multitask. For instance, if you have a toddler or work in an industry that will have you on the go, these are used as a more discreet way to pump in several settings.

MILK SUPPLY

As your baby gets a little older and you possibly return to work, to continue to match your baby's needs, you will need to set a nursing and/or pumping schedule to keep up your milk supply. Your body produces milk based on demand, therefore as you reduce your sessions you will also be reducing your supply. In contrast the more you nurse and/or pump the more you produce to meet the appetite of your baby. Milk is produced based on stimulation. A good rule of thumb is to never go more than 5 hours without nursing or pumping. Doing so inherently tells your body to slow down production. This rule also applies to newborns, your newborn should not go more than 5 hours without a feeding.

It can be hard to gauge how much milk you should be pumping. As a reference point, if you plan to pump exclusively, you should plan to produce on average 25-35 ounces of milk in 24 hours. Don't expect these numbers during the first week of breastfeeding, you will need to gradually work up to these numbers. In my case, my doula suggested that I waited 6 weeks to establish a good milk supply and latch before pumping. I know the ability to follow this commitment varies depending on your maternity leave and career demands, but this did indeed work for me. I was able to use the milk saver to catch leaking milk during the first few weeks. I stored this milk as little ice cubes and was able to throw them into the bottle when we were ready to introduce a bottle. We introduced a bottle around 6-8 weeks but very infrequently. I would suggest getting a bottle that is engineered to mimic the breast. We didn't experience any issues going between bottle and breast.

At 8 weeks, I began pumping at night, during the early morning hours, and pumped the remaining milk after a nursing session. This can vary depending on your baby's sleep pattern or appetite. The key is to empty often. So, once you have nursed your little one before bed or a nap, you would pump whatever milk remains once your baby is asleep. It's important to do this sooner rather than later to give your body ample time to produce more milk before their next feeding.

I know I'm making all this sound easy, and I know every day will not be so, but hopefully, this information will guide you through those days and help you make more informed choices.

I would suggest that you set some goals on how to save milk. I started with saving one bottle a day and worked my way up to two bottles a day. Milk supplements also helped not just for producing more breastmilk, but for producing thicker and more filling milk. This allowed me to save more because she was full, with less. Take full advantage of your mornings because due to am hormone release, it's common to produce more milk in the morning. Use this time to store extra milk, your baby will more than likely leave a good amount of milk to be pumped. Also, take notice of an overproducing left or right breast. If you notice that your baby favors one breast over the other, be sure to empty the other to avoid clogged ducts or a reduction in production.

Breastfeeding is a commitment full of rewards. I can attest to experiencing these benefits. Initially, I felt my uterus contracting each time I breastfed, this allowed my uterus to revert to its natural size. I also lost all my baby weight in under 12 months! I thought my weight loss had become stagnant around 5 months but between 6-8 months my weight loss picked up with her growth spurts.

The hormonal changes associated with breastfeeding helped establish the nurturing and bonding needed to establish a deep connection and desire to make it through those long days and nights. Each of those tough moments was accompanied by mommy's milk and, I can say, she came to notice my hard days. As a toddler now, she knows when to walk over and warm me up with a kiss or simply lay on my chest. We're so in tune some days, it's like we have our own language. I can typically meet her needs within minutes solely through her body language.

As much as I enjoyed breastfeeding, I reached a point, after 6 teeth and 12 months of feeling chained to my breast pump, where I was ready to part ways with this chapter of motherhood. I missed falling asleep for the night without the anxiety of pumping to keep my milk supply steady. At 12 months, and after being quarantined to our home during a pandemic for 2 ½ months, I stopped pumping. There were countless reasons to stop, my baby had become a crawler and walker and was getting into everything. I could no longer pump while she laid still on her tummy or back. She was sleeping less and less during the day. Why was I pumping? We no longer had childcare. Plus, I was nearing the end of the duration I had planned to breastfeed. I had originally planned to nurse for 6 months then extended it to 12 months after realizing I preferred breastfeeding over choosing a powdered formula to trust. It made more sense for me to wait until 12 months when Formula was no longer needed, and we could switch to whole milk or almond milk.

At 12 months, I was back to nursing exclusively although I tried to limit my nursing to 3-4 sessions a day. These sessions were linked to naps and bedtime. This is common since the hardest sessions to stop are typically the first morning sessions, naps, and bedtime. After breastfeeding for 14 months, I slowly cut back on our nursing sessions to the point where I was only nursing for bed and naps.

The easiest way for us was through distractions. We visited the grandparents for a long weekend, she was so distracted each morning, I was able to change the am routine. I started brushing her teeth first thing in the morning and then it was straight to breakfast with a cup of almond milk. The final challenge was getting her to sleep without nursing. This is where you will need family and/or a partner to step in. My sister stepped in on a week-long visit to help me stop nursing. She started with naps and transitioned to bedtime. After she left, my partner stepped in to finish the next couple of nights I was not nursing during bedtime. Within 3-4 days, we were done with nursing. I must say that those first few days of pulling the plug are a bit unbearable when your baby is crying out for the one thing that puts them to sleep with ease. But stay the course, you'll both eventually get there! Of course, you will miss this time with your baby too. But eventually, it will be time to reclaim your body, Mama, and it will be so good to close this chapter knowing you accomplished what you set out to do.

I've put together a breastfeeding checklist to help you achieve your breastfeeding goals. You've got this Mama!

BREASTFEEDING CHECKLIST:

- [ ] Milk collector (For leaking breast)
- [ ] 7-10 nursing bras in different styles
- [ ] Pumping bras or bras with add-on pumping accessory
- [ ] Reusable Nursing pads
- [ ] A few stylish, comfortable pairs of pajamas with easy nursing access
- [ ] Nursing tops or simple tops with easy nursing access
- [ ] Breast Pump
- [ ] Replacement parts for pump
- [ ] Sanitization spray for breast pump
- [ ] Milk supplements
- [ ] Heating pad
- [ ] Night light for late-night nursing
- [ ] Cozy nursing chair in the nursery
- [ ] Nursing cover
- [ ] Find a lactation consultant.

- ☐ Join a mommy group like La Leche League

8 HOLISTIC WAYS TO INCREASE YOUR MILK SUPPLY

1. Lactation teas and treats
2. Pumping after each nursing session, to signal your body to produce more milk.
3. More skin to skin. Lay baby on your bare chest with only a diaper on to increase the production of breastmilk-producing hormones like oxytocin.
4. Do not supplement with formula or skip feedings.
5. Stay hydrated! Breastfeeding requires you to drink more water than the 11 cups suggested for women.
6. Eat foods that increase your milk supply - oats, leafy greens, almonds, ginger, brown rice, salmon, asparagus, eggs, sweet potatoes, sardines.
7. Try supplements and herbs - blessed thistle, red raspberry tea, fenugreek, Brewer's yeast, Moringa, Nettle, vervain.
8. Most importantly, nurse on demand! Give that baby what they want!

BREASTFEEDING AFFIRMATIONS:

- Breast milk is liquid gold.
- Breastfeeding helps protect my baby.
- My breastmilk was created for my baby.
- Breastfeeding creates an undeniable bond between me and my baby.

- Every day will not be perfect and, that's okay.
- I trust my feelings and insights as a mother.
- My breast milk continuously adapts as my baby grows to meet his or her changing nutritional needs.
- It is okay for me to make and take time for myself. I understand that I need to be healthy in my mind, body, and spirit to provide for my little ones.
- Some days are tough, others come with ease.
- My baby and I are always learning and growing together.
- I can provide all the nourishment my baby needs.
- There is nothing better than time spent nourishing my baby.
- It is ok if my baby nurses frequently.
- I won't give up; this will get easier.

10

ESTABLISHING A NEW NORMAL

We have covered a lot of ground on our journey through pregnancy, birthing prep, meeting your baby, postpartum, and breastfeeding, and now we are establishing our new normal. While there are days when I miss the simple things like cuddling all day with my newborn while being disconnected from the outside world, there are also days when I found maternity leave and breastfeeding to be very isolating. As you settle into the state of healing and rest, mixed with the nonstop act of breastfeeding, you will become a bit stagnant and have a hard time getting outside. Many new moms initially feel a bit of anxiety when it comes to driving or going out into the world with their delicate newborn and healing body. I had to be intentional about establishing a routine that involved weekly outings to leave the house and socialize. This helped me initiate a routine, discover the ins and outs of getting us out of the house on time, and how to properly prepare for baby incidents.

Here is a list of things to do on maternity leave to get you and your baby out of the house:

- Playdates
- Mommy dates with/or without baby

- Lunch dates to visit partner or family
- Mommy and Me fitness classes
- Grandparents' house
- Shopping centers, malls, and markets
- Infant movie matinee
- Eco-friendly nail salons
- Visit museums
- Visit botanical gardens
- Breastfeeding Center
- Library story-time activities

You can most definitely use this list for just yourself, as a new mommy, know that you will need time to recharge because things can become overwhelming while adjusting to the new demands of motherhood. In addition to the list above, go to a spa. Get facials, massages, have no nursing days, if need be, take the long way to the coffee shop, window shop, and do whatever you need to do to reclaim some of your independence and recharge.

As much as I love working out, this is the one time in my life where I strongly suggest taking it slowly. I started working out again right around my 6-week appointment. Once I was cleared by my midwife, I gradually started walking on the treadmill or riding a stationary bike in our apartment gym again. I would often wear my baby girl or let her sleep in her pram. I also joined a local Mommy and Me yoga class. I was able to get reacquainted with my body and try out positions to see how they felt since giving birth. This was a safe space. It was typically understood that you may be late or need to nurse during class, and all scenarios were welcome. The instructor was great at reading the room and knew when to switch to more baby attention or just hold the baby while mommy focused on her downward dog.

At 3 months postpartum, I joined a mommy stroller workout that was exactly what I needed. I was out of the house every weekday by 9 a.m. to join a group of fellow new moms on maternity leave. We jogged, exchanged mom tricks, found a shoulder to lean on, and always had someone cheering us on in all aspects of life. These activities brought light to some of my darkest postpartum days. I found it beneficial to be around women going through similar situations, especially finding a community that is a judgment-free zone surrounding breastfeeding. You will find that breastfeeding can cause some isolation during this time, especially if you are dealing with intergenerational trauma with your family. You may feel pressured to breastfeed behind closed doors. I recall having to often step away from family events, social settings, and dinner tables mid-conversation, to tend to my new baby. Do what is best for you. If you prefer privacy, then take it, if you are comfortable where you are, do that too. However, it is that you choose to take care of yourself and your baby, I suggest that new mommies join some activities that welcome your current lifestyle and get that dopamine and endorphins flowing, you will thank me later.

Since every mom's delivery experience and healing is different, please be sure to be cleared by your health professional before engaging in physical activity. It is completely normal to have a weak bladder or leakage after giving birth, so take it easy with jumping and running. Beginning physical activity before you are healed can cause more harm and prolonged bleeding. Also, ask your healthcare or therapeutic professional about Diastasis Recti. It's a gap in between your right and left abdominal wall muscles from your belly expanding to carry a baby. This gap can result in a rounded, protruding belly "pooch," if it does not heal correctly. Some exercises can be used to repair the separation. Physical therapy and core-specific Pilates can also be great resources for correcting this without creating more damage.

Postpartum depression is another thing to look out for in mommies of newborns. I hope that by following a postpartum plan, you will manage this transitional time so you can emerge stronger, happier, and feeling whole. Part of this plan is to develop a tribe you can rely on for help on this new journey. This support will allow you to evolve into a confident mother who can trust her instincts. This time can be coupled with doubt, uncertainty, and new mom anxiety. The first few months, even years, can be overwhelming. Women come into motherhood already juggling so much. Add to that your body changes and hormonal imbalance, and you are going to need all the physical and emotional help you can get. The newborn workload is temporary, but you will need a tribe to remind you of this throughout this process. As your baby gets older and gains more independence, you will notice your workload becoming a little lighter by the day. Yes, believe me when I say a day will come when there will be fewer diaper changes, more self-feedings, enhanced personality, and more giggles! Until that day comes, rely on your tribe for support and companionship. You will reemerge and look back on this time with satisfaction, knowing that you were able to morph through some significant, major changes.

While there are difficulties and challenges every new mother must face, it is my goal that by shedding light on these issues, you can move through your challenges with the power of knowledge and less uncertainty.

Embrace your body, it can create life! It can and will recover from whatever birth experience you've encountered. The hormones will balance out as your uterus shrinks back down to its original size. Expect some tears and some anxiety associated with caring for your baby and, if you feel you are experiencing more than baby blues and light sadness, please speak to a therapist and seek help. The hormonal imbalance experienced after giving birth is serious, so if at any time you feel that you cannot lift your spirits and you are feeling more misunderstood than supported, please contact someone. It is courageous to identify this problem and respond accordingly to the health of you, your baby, and your family.

Here's a Postpartum Depression Checklist to help you identify if you need to seek additional support:

DO YOU . . .

- Have trouble sleeping?
- Find you're exhausted most of the time?
- Notice a decrease in your appetite?
- Worry about little things that never used to bother you?
- Wonder if you'll ever have time to yourself again?
- Think your children would be better off without you?

- Worry that your partner will get tired of you feeling this way?
- Snap at your partner and children over everything?
- Think everyone else is a better mother than you are?
- Cry over the slightest thing?
- No longer enjoy the things you used to enjoy?
- Isolate yourself from your friends and neighbors?
- Fear leaving the house or being alone?
- Have anxiety attacks?
- Have unexplained anger?
- Do you have difficulty concentrating?
- Think something else is wrong with you or your marriage?
- Feel like you will always feel this way and never get better?

If you answered yes to more than three (3) of these questions you may be experiencing postpartum depression. According to National data, 20% of women experience postpartum depression. For Black women, the risk is twice as high while remaining less likely to seek help. Due to the mental health stigma and the agenda of this only being a joyous time, the numbers may be lagging tremendously, because it's not easy prioritizing your mental health after waiting 9 months for your new baby. But I assure you that many new moms are experiencing these symptoms too, so there's no need to feel embarrassed or to suffer in silence. If the suggestions for adjusting to your new normal don't uplift you, please seek professional support.

Postpartum hit me hard. I was not diagnosed with postpartum depression, although at each post-natal appointment my questionnaire responses were considered red flags. I was never referred to or contacted by a professional. Unfortunately, the American maternity care system is not currently set up to provide immediate mental health support or resources. New resources are being created every day by new mothers, such as yourself, that see the lack of support for mothers during this transitional period. I did eventually start regular therapy sessions. Motherhood has a way of shedding light on childhood traumas and highlighting things that are long overdue to be unpacked. These sessions helped me to establish boundaries with parents and other care providers, address my needs to my partner, and to set expectations for motherhood.

For me, I struggled mostly with losing my independence. I missed being able to get up and go. The idea of taking time to myself was always bombarded by a long list of other tasks that would always outweigh my desire to take some time away, or from mom-guilt for not doing those tasks. My energy was low from long nights and early mornings. At times, it felt that the preparation to get away was more than I was able to do. I wanted everything to be perfect before I left and when I returned. This caused me an overwhelming amount of anxiety because it's simply not possible. I had to learn to let go and to allow others to be the caregivers and support me as I took time away to recharge. The age-old saying is true, *you cannot pour from an empty cup.*

Mom-guilt is real. It's fostered by society's never-ending expectations of mothers and women. We often get these expectations from social media, family and friends, and work settings about what moms should be like or what they should be doing.

It can be tough to not let these feelings sneak in especially when you need some time to yourself. Remind yourself that you are enough. That it is ok to take breaks and time away for yourself. Childbirth and motherhood are huge undertakings, they will take a lot out of you. But for you to feel complete, you must learn to step away even when you would rather hold your baby all day. Spend the day pampering yourself or taking a walk alone. It may seem strange at first but, before you know it, you will realize that remembering who you are will make you a better mother.

Remember that the journey to motherhood can be such a joyful and blissful experience for every woman, including Black women, and I want you to have that! And you can, if you are still in the process of trying or thinking of becoming pregnant. If you have already been there, it's not too late, you can share your newly acquired knowledge with the women who will follow you into motherhood.

Every time a Black baby is born, a Black mom is born. This should never be taken lightly. Black women are the backbones of our families and keeping that backbone healthy and stable is a key component to our communities' success.

We know that the resources and conversations are lacking in our communities. We have the power to pass down knowledge to one another. Each time I hear the statistics surrounding maternal and infant mortality rates, I know we can no longer afford to postpone these conversations. We need our Black women armed with the necessary information to make choices for more positive outcomes. These positive outcomes can look like many things:

- Feeling empowered after birth
- Giving your baby a birth experience, you did not have
- More examples in your family for breastfeeding
- Advocating for ourselves in hospital settings
- More homebirths
- Hiring Doulas
- Working with a midwife
- Choosing providers that look like you
- Healthy newborns who are born ready to latch
- Fewer interventions
- Proper healing following birth
- Connected birth experiences
- Longer breastfeeding periods

BLACK MOM AFFIRMATIONS:

- I am raising beautiful Black children who will change the world.
- Being a Black mom is my superpower.
- I become a more confident mother with each new day.
- I trust my maternal instincts.
- I will take care of myself and show up for my children and family.
- Every day will not be perfect and that is ok.
- There is magic and power in creating new Black life.
- Sometimes being a good mother means letting go. Everything will not go as planned.
- I am my ancestor's wildest dreams.

- I deserve to take care of myself – mind, body, and soul.
- Cherish these moments because this time will not last forever.
- Even strong Black women need to rest and reset. I give myself space to do just that.
- I am my child's life-long teacher.
- I set the tone for my family's day. I am a vital part of our productivity.

An unmedicated birth may not be an option for all but, I do believe it's certainly an option for more Black women who are having them today. We can say no to interventions and trust in our abilities. We control our bodies, and, with preparation, it will support us through anything. Suffering is not a requirement of the Black maternal identity. Instead, we should equip ourselves with our ancestors and their instincts to act, letting go of the passive relationship we have with our bodies instead of being leaders of them. Our ancestors have birthed nations with pride and strength. They spread knowledge and supported one another throughout the process of birth, postpartum, and breastfeeding. They came together in villages and carried each new mother through this rite of passage with cultivated support and love that is missing from the modern Black birth experience.

More connected birth experiences first require desire and intention. I hope this book brings forth the desire to prepare and educate yourself for birth and that you move with intention throughout the entire birth experience. Join me in reducing

Black maternal and infant mortality rates, I cannot make the change without you Black birthing mommas.

I hope this book encouraged a deeper dive into the Black maternal history in this country and shows every woman, especially Black women, the meaning behind our choices and what happens when we birth our babies in rooms that are not making our well-being or our history a priority. If you only take one thing away from this book, let it be that every choice matters. Who you choose to be in your birthing room matters. Who you choose as your provider matters. Where you choose to birth matters. What you choose to eat matters. How active you are matters. The mindset you choose matters. It all matters!

If you need more support, you can reach me at @1NicoleBailey on Instagram or email me at Nicole@bodybellysoul.com. For more resources and continued pregnancy and new mom support, check out my website www.BodyBellySoul.com.

ACKNOWLEDGMENTS

I would like to start by thanking the man who chose this journey of parenthood with me, my ambitious partner, and the love of my life. Thank you for pushing me and standing by me every step of the way. I shared my vision and ideas of birth with you, and you embodied them as your own. We share a strong desire to uplift our community and we start with our family each day.

My daughter, Alexandria Bailey, I love you more than anything in this world. You have shown me love in its purest form. Thank you for choosing me to be your mother. I am more than proud to pass down the same legacy from your grandmother to you. You must now carry the torch.

I would also like to thank my parents for showing me the power of discipline and resilience. You gave me the courage to birth the way I knew was possible.

Thank you to my younger sister for showing up in her new role as Titi. For being a part of our village and supporting us through the many transitions.

Huge thank you to my mommy tribe! Sky, Alize, Jade, and Althea – I do not know where I would be without each of you. You all constantly reminded me of what I was capable of and showed real transparency surrounding your birthing experiences. I do not take this lightly. I am forever grateful to have joined this lifelong tribe with each other. Let's raise more Black Queens.

Sis-cousins – Atilah, Oriana, Tarol, and Victoria. Thank you for encouraging me, reminding me to choose myself, and pushing me outside of my comfort zone.

Fatima Abdallah, our Doula, thank you for prepping my family for the most beautiful birth experience we could have ever imagined. Your gentle spirit was a guide.

GW Midwives – Thank you to the midwives for creating a safe space for mothers to birth the way they want.

Amma, developmental editor, and momma – Thank you for being there every step of the way writing this book. You showed patience and helped bring my ideas to light.

To all the Black mothers reading this book, thank you for allowing me to share my story and give hope to more positive birth stories. We can reduce Black maternal and infant mortality together.

SOURCES CITED

"A Brief History of Black Midwifery in the US." DTI, May 1, 2019. https://doulatrainingsinternational.com/brief-history-black-midwifery-us/

Abedin, Shahren. "Hypnobirthing Classes, How It Works, Methods, and More." WebMD. WebMD, June 15, 2010. https://www.webmd.com/baby/features/hypnobirthing-calmer-natural-childbirth

Ani, Amanishakete. "C-Section and Racism: 'Cutting' to the Heart of the Issue for Black Women and Families." *Journal of African American Studies* 19, no. 4 (2015): 343-61. https://doi.org/10.1007/s12111-015-9310-4

Bjarnadottir, Adda. "11 Benefits of Breastfeeding for Both Mom and Baby." Healthline. Healthline Media, August 13, 2020. https://www.healthline.com/nutrition/11-benefits-of-breastfeeding.

"Black Mothers and C-Section Births: Commoditized Oppression and Existential Violence." Afrometrics. 9/18/2020. http://www.afrometrics.org/

research-based-news/black-mothers-and-C-section-births-commoditized-oppression-and-existential-violence.

Buckley, Sarah J. Executive Summary. In Hormonal Physiology of Childbearing: Evidence and Implications for Women, Babies, and Maternity Care. Washington, D.C.: Childbirth Connection Programs, National Partnership for Women & Families, January 2015. https://www.nationalpartnership.org/our-work/resources/health-care/maternity/hormonal-physiology-of-childbearing-exec-summary.pdf

Carmon, Irin. "For Eugenic Sterilization Victims, Belated Justice." MSNBC. NBCUniversal News Group, October 1, 2020. http://www.msnbc.com/all/eugenic-sterilization-victims-belated-justice.

"Choice or Coercion - The Biography of Norplant." Episode, n.d.

"Evidence on: Doulas." Evidence-Based Birth®, August 12, 2019. https://evidencebasedbirth.com/the-evidence-for-doulas/

Freeman, Andrea. Skimmed: Breastfeeding, Race, and Injustice. S.l.: Stanford University Press, 2021.

Freeman, Andrea. "Unmothering Black Women: Formula Feeding as an Incident of Slavery." Hastings Law Journal 69, no. 6 (2018): 1546-1606. http://www.hastingslawjournal.org/wp-content/uploads/Freeman-69.6.pdf

Garippo, Gina. "5 Medications You May Receive During Labor and Delivery." Healthgrades. Healthgrades, February

13, 2020. https://www.healthgrades.com/right-care/pregnancy/5-medications-you-may-receive-during-labor-and-delivery.

Genevieve, Howland. "The Mama Natural Week by Week Guide to Pregnancy & Childbirth." Mama Natural, March 12, 2018. https://www.mamanatural.com/book/week-by-week-guide-pregnancy-childbirth/.

"Having a Doula - What Are the Benefits?" American Pregnancy Association, March 10, 2021. https://americanpregnancy.org/healthy-pregnancy/labor-and-birth/having-a-doula-616

"Her Holistic Path – 5 mistakes to avoid when planning your birth." Broadcast, n.d.

"Her Holistic Path – How I had a Painless natural birth." Broadcast, n.d.

"Her Holistic Path – What's the Difference between Doula, Midwife and OB/GYN." Broadcast, n.d.

"Honoring the Legacy Black Lay Midwives of the South." Black Then, March 20, 2020. https://blackthen.com/honoring-the-legacy-black-lay-midwives-of-the-south/

"How Formula Milk Firms Target Mothers Who Can Least Afford It." The Guardian. Guardian News and Media, February 27, 2018. https://www.theguardian.com/lifeandstyle/2018/feb/27/formula-milk-companies-target-poor-mothers-breastfeeding/

Johnson, Kimberly Ann. "The Fourth Trimester: A Postpartum Guide to Healing Your Body, Balancing Your Emotions, and Restoring Your Vitality." Amazon. Shambhala, 2017. https://www.amazon.com/Fourth-Trimester-Postpartum-Balancing-Restoring/dp/1611804000.

Kelly, Djenaba Dioum. "The Power of Traditional African Healing Methods." Chopra. Chopra, January 14, 2016. https://chopra.com/articles/the-power-of-traditional-african-healing-methods.

OBOS Pregnancy & Birth Contributors | April 7. "Questions to Ask When Selecting a Doctor or Midwife." Our Bodies Ourselves, May 12, 2017. https://www.ourbodiesourselves.org/book-excerpts/health-article/questions-to-ask-when-selecting-a-doctor-or-midwife/.

Oyelana, Olabisi, Joyce Kamanzi, and Solina Richter. "A Critical Look at Exclusive Breastfeeding in Africa: Through the Lens of Diffusion of Innovation Theory." *International Journal of Africa Nursing Sciences* 14 (2021): 100267. https://doi.org/10.1016/j.ijans.2020.100267.

Person. "Finding Healing in the Spiritual Practices of Our Ancestors." Shondaland. Shondaland, September 11, 2019. https://www.shondaland.com/live/body/a28989067/finding-healing-i-spiritual-practices-ancestors/.

Roberts, Dorothy E. *Killing the Black Body: Race, Reproduction, and the Meaning of Liberty*. New York: Vintage Book, a division of Penguin Random House LLC, 2017.

Rochman, Bonnie. "C-Sections on the Rise, Especially for Black Moms." Time. Time, December 20, 2010. https://healthland.time.com/2010/12/20/c-sections-on-the-rise-especially-for-black-moms.

Rooks, Judith P. "The History of Midwifery." Our Bodies Ourselves, June 14, 2016. https://www.ourbodiesourselves.org/book-excerpts/health-article/history-of-midwifery/.

Schwartz, Marie Jenkins. "Birthing a Slave: Motherhood and Medicine in the Antebellum South." Amazon. Harvard University Press, 2009. https://www.amazon.com/Birthing-Slave-Motherhood-Medicine-Antebellum/dp/0674034929.

Schwartz, Marie Jenkins. *Birthing a Slave: Motherhood and Medicine in the Antebellum South*. Cambridge, MA: Harvard University Press, 2009.

Suzanne Schlosberg. "33 Reasons to Exercise Now." Parents, April 23, 2014. https://www.parents.com/pregnancy/my-body/fitness/ten-reasons-to-get-off-the-couch/.

Timmons, Jessica. "Chiropractor While Pregnant: Benefits." Healthline. Healthline Media, August 2, 2016. https://www.healthline.com/health/pregnancy/chiropractor-while-pregnant.

"The Cascade of Intervention." Homepage. http://www.childbirthconnection.org/maternity-care/cascade-of-intervention/.

"Women in D.C. Face Obstacles at Every Step of Pregnancy and Childbirth." Community of Hope. Accessed April 23, 2021. https://www.communityofhopedc.org/news-events/women-dc-face-obstacles-every-step-pregnancy-and-childbirth.

ABOUT THE AUTHOR

"You give birth the same way that you live"

Nicole Bailey graduated from the University of North Carolina at Greensboro with a bachelor's degree in public health and a minor in nutrition and went on to attend Drexel School of Medicine to obtain a master's in clinical trial organization and management. Nicole has worked in the clinical trial industry for over 10 years and has always had a passion for health, research, and history. She developed her knowledge of women and the birth process by completing training as a doula, studying global quality maternal and newborn care at Yale University, and breastfeeding support at Stanford University. After writing this book, she created an extended online platform called *Body Belly Soul*, with the intent of guiding Black mothers towards primal, powerful, and peaceful birth experiences. Her mission is to strive for more connected birthing experiences among Black mothers. Together with her husband, they have dedicated their lives to closing the health and wealth gap in the Black community. They reside in Washington, D.C. with their daughter.